The Enigma of Hastings

Edwin Tetlow

The Enigma of Hastings

PETER OWEN · LONDON

ISBN 0 7206 0003 0

PETER OWEN LIMITED
20 Holland Park Avenue
London W11 3QU

First British Commonwealth edition 1974
© Edwin Tetlow 1974

Printed in Great Britain by
Bristol Typesetting Co Ltd
Barton Manor - St Philips
Bristol

Contents

Illustrations

Foreword

This work is the outcome of well over half a lifetime, almost 50 years in fact, spent in intermittent but permanent dalliance with the hazy story of the lives and times of Harold Godwinson, King of England, and his conqueror, William, Duke of Normandy. My interest in the topic was first stirred when as a boy I chanced upon a copy of Lord Bulwer-Lytton's great historical novel, *Harold, Last of the Saxon Kings.* The book is theatrical, and morbid in its theme, but it is extraordinarily thrilling and evocative. After reading it several times I was inspired to make a study of the Conquest a hobby to be pursued whenever possible during a demanding career as a reporter, war correspondent, foreign correspondent and writer of books.

A twentieth-century Englishman cannot but feel kinship with Harold and William and the thousands of unknown men who fought for and against them and, by so doing, created a close-knit and enviable island kingdom which, for all its faults, is one to which a man need not be ashamed to belong. In my case, the bond is more than ordinarily personal because, it seems, an ancestor who provided the family name (originally Tete-de-Loup) was thieving, poaching and fighting as an Anglo-Saxon guerilla in the shaded world of Sherwood Forest not long after the Battle of Hastings – tormenting and dodging his Norman pursuers and getting himself posted on the trees in placards under the ignominious symbol of outlawry, the wolf's head, as a man wanted dead or alive by his lords. There is no record of his doom, but his family fear the worst.

Scholars and specialists have written, often with brilliance and authority, upon many aspects of the Conquest. But nobody, so far as I know, has done what I have tried to do – to write a factual account in the manner of the reporter and war correspondent, seeking to produce a narrative which can serve as a text for accuracy and conciseness without, one hopes, losing wide appeal. Above all, I have tried to dissect and sift the pro-Norman propaganda which

9

has always dominated the subject, so that a reader may be inclined to think twice before accepting whatever he has been told or has read previously.

My heartfelt gratitude is acknowledged, and hereby offered, to my wife, K., who for forty years not only aided my research but produced invaluable material on her own initiative and as a culminating service checked the final manuscript. I wish also to record my debt to my friend, Niels Nørlund, of Langerød, Denmark, for making available a treasured copy of *Trelleborg* (Copenhagen, 1948), written by his father, the late P. Nørlund, and translated from the Danish by J. R. B. Gosney. Similarly Professor Michel de Bouard of the University of Caen (Normandy) is thanked for his willing and effective co-operation, and A. E. Stevenson, of Battle, is also thanked for the use of a fascinating analysis, 'Where was Malfosse? The End of the Battle of Hastings,' written by C. T. Chevallier as chairman of the Battle and District Historical Society. And I wish to express appreciation to Bethy Withycombe for translating into comprehensible English some tortuous and obscure medieval Latin.

Finally, a tribute is due to the New York Public Library. No demand was too troublesome for the staff of this splendid institution, and its shelves and archives rarely failed to produce a desired work or manuscript, no matter how recondite.

Alligerville, New York, and   EDWIN TETLOW
South Leigh, Oxfordshire.
Summer, 1973

An Embroidered Tale

One of the most tantalizing political-military mysteries in 1,000 years of world history concerns the Norman Conquest of England. Everyone knows the year of the brief and bloody battle which – to the surprise even of the winner in 1066 – gave without further military ado the misty and alluring island kingdom to Duke William of Normandy; and everybody save the most ill-disposed has some time felt a pang of pity for the man who lost, King Harold, last of the Anglo-Saxon royal line, who according to legend was struck down with an arrow in his eye late in the afternoon of Saturday, 14 October, while still heroically smiting out for England and himself, along with a dwindled band of faithful warriors engaged in a now hopeless struggle against the alien invader. Many who feel stirring within them a kinship with the lost Anglo-Saxon kingdom despise the unsporting trick which William they say, played when he told his archers to release their light but sharply-pointed arrows in a lofty arc so that they would fall behind the English shields and, as with the luckless Harold, pierce the defenders from an unexpected direction.

But was it really like that?

Some facts about the battle and the Conquest are to be accepted without cavil, of course, because they are founded upon unchallengeable contemporary documents such as royal, legal and religious writs and edicts and, above all, the painstaking entries in the Domesday Book where the particulars about every strip of inhabited land in the country were recorded in 1086 at William's command. In many instances their condition before and after the battle of Hastings could be compared. But there is much uncertainty about such vital matters as the background and timing of William's hazardous but successful venture, Harold's role in the affair before he became king and during his reign of ten months, the relationship between William and others who had covetous eyes upon England in 1066, and even what happened during the battle itself. The story is befogged by legend, lie, propaganda and, in many of its aspects, by lack of acceptable evidence. The most frustrating circumstance of all is that almost all the items of unofficial evidence – those which may be described as 'the juicy bits' – come down to us from one side only. So we must beware of accepting wholesale the stories of the Conquest given by Norman chroniclers, troubadours and sycophants, who could scarcely be expected to write or otherwise compose anything at all disagreeable to William, the winner and their patron. Most of them were operating at second hand, after the event, and we may be sure that their relayed and delayed tales would lose nothing in the telling. Indeed, since human nature seems not to have changed much in a thousand years, many of these reporters probably went out of their way to outdo their contemporaries in decorating the facts. The practice is still common today.

There exists, to be sure, one incomparable unofficial memento of the period in the Bayeux Tapestry. Yet even this creation must be viewed with serious suspicion as regards its factual accuracy, since its purpose was undoubtedly to provide, admittedly with great artistry and often in stunning detail, a picture story of what the Normans would have everybody believe happened. The priceless production is about 75 yards long and 20 inches wide and its eight colours have faded during the passage of more than nine centuries into soft and highly appealing shades. It is thought to have been embroidered by humble English seamstresses engaged and sustained by Duke William's half-brother, Bishop Odo of Bayeux, and directed by authors and designers of rare talent, who cleverly fulfilled their mission of producing for a mostly illiterate public one of the world's early strip-cartoons, spiced with enough blood and thunder and ribaldry (in some sections of its lower border) to attract the interest and attention of those to whom it was meant to carry a message but not the truth. The precise date of its making is not known but nobody now doubts that this must have been within living memory of the invasion of 1066 and the purported events occurring in the years immediately preceding it.

We shall be doing well to admire the Tapestry but to mistrust it. Its clear purpose is to justify William's assault upon England and to magnify his triumph in carrying it off. The first 30 of the

80 or so panels into which the Tapestry may conveniently be divided for viewing purposes is devoted to proving, with much circumstantial detail, that William had every right to cross the English Channel with his powerful force to strike a usurping Harold off his throne. This is the theme of all Norman propaganda about the Conquest, and the basis for the justification is depicted with emphasis in the Tapestry. It is a visit which Harold is supposed to have made to William a few years before 1066 on an order from Edward the Confessor, the reigning King of England, to confirm a promise made earlier to William that he was to succeed to the throne if (as happened) Edward died without an heir.

This is an unlikely tale indeed. For one thing, the throne was not Edward's to give away in such a fashion. In Anglo-Saxon times the prerogative of deciding the succession had always lain with the Witan, or Great Council, composed of the lay and clerical leaders of the kingdom. Secondly, for more than a decade before 1066 Harold was the most powerful man in the country next to the king, and everything he did officially was obviously of importance. Consequently, such a momentous event as an official visit to Normandy on behalf of the king, whatever its purpose, would certainly have been recorded somewhere. The fact is that not one word about this visit was written anywhere in England at or near the time it is supposed by the Normans to have happened (1064), so far as has been discovered during the succeeding nine centuries.

Perhaps the most convincing evidence against the visit ever having happened, at least in the form which William's propagandists would have us accept, is that not one of the several versions of the Anglo-Saxon Chronicle, a fascinating annual record of the principal events affecting the kingdom between 60 BC and AD 1135 contains a single word about it. This unique diary is the solid foundation upon which has been built the story of early England. Its entries are terse and sometimes apparently irrelevant or incomplete – here and there maddeningly so – but its veracity is not to be doubted. It was not kept in the customary Latin but in the vernacular Anglo-Saxon by monks in various monasteries, notably at Abingdon, Peterborough and Worcester, who probably passed copies of their writings from one to another. Each scribe could thus learn what was being written by his fellows and, as was often done, add something to his own record about events close to home with which he was familiar. It is inconceivable that the Chronicles should simply

have ignored any embassy by Earl Harold – although they might
not have troubled themselves about an informal journey across the
Channel such as a hunting trip to Normandy. In particular, the
Abingdon version of the Anglo-Saxon Chronicle should certainly
be expected to record so damaging an event as a sacred oath of
allegiance made by Harold to William while in Normandy, for this
version was hostile to the House of Godwin, of which Harold was
now the head, and its scribe would surely have pounced upon the
sensational news of a renunciatory pledge by Harold. In fact, neither
he nor any of his fellow scribes found anything worth their attention
to record for 1064.

The extraordinary minuteness with which the Tapestry describes
the visit and the taking of the oath can be explained if one accepts
the theory that the Tapestry is basically a vehicle of propaganda.
A mass of circumstantial evidence adds verisimilitude to any story.
In this instance, such auxiliary details would be particularly useful,
indeed essential, to the Normans in 'planting' a story in an era
when the common man was infinitely more credulous and superstitious than he later became. To him an oath was a fearful thing
and any man who broke one was considered doomed, so that a
concocted story making Harold a perjuror would have a powerful
propagandist impact upon the populace.

The purpose was nothing less than to make a *post facto* justification of the invasion and seizure of an independent kingdom.
William's publicity agents, directed by Bishop Odo, set an example
in embroidering the facts (in more senses than one) which was to
be followed with improved means by later tyrants, even so recent a
one as Adolf Hitler who similarly employed the talents of Joseph
Goebbels to warrant his successful invasion of Austria and
Czechoslovakia, and his ultimately unsuccessful one against Poland.
The creators of the Tapestry would seem to be vulnerable to a
charge of using what became known in the twentieth century as
'the technique of the big lie'. But in one respect at least they balked
at going the whole way. The Tapestry avoids mentioning the specific
terms of the oath Harold purportedly swore before William. The
inscription on the panel depicting this highly dramatic occurrence
runs: Where Harold made an oath to Duke William (*Ubi Harold
sacramentum fecit Willelmo duci*).

A pertinent question instantly arises. If Harold swore to reserve
the throne of England for William, why does the Tapestry not say

so, instead of talking merely about 'an oath'? One reason for this apparent lapse may be that Odo intended the Tapestry to go on permanent view at his church at Bayeux and did not feel it politic to have so flagrant a lie proclaimed so blatantly. Perhaps he felt that the Norman purpose could be more adroitly served by leaving it to less 'official' and less obtrusive chroniclers to fill in the story. This theory is stimulated by an extraordinary performance in the matter by William of Poitiers, an ardent admirer of Duke William and a propagandist who (as we shall see) served his master well, if sycophantically. William of Poitiers was early in his career a soldier. Then he became a priest, served for a time as William's chaplain and eventually became Archdeacon of Lisieux. His version of the terms of the oath said to have been sworn by Harold is so pre-posterous as to confirm in the mind of any independent observer the falsity of the whole story. In the course of a flowery account of the Conquest which he wrote in 1071 he claimed that 'as is testified by the most truthful and most honourable men who were there present' Harold swore that :

1. He would be the representative of Duke William at the court of his lord, King Edward, as long as the king lived;

2. He would use all his influence and wealth to ensure that after the death of King Edward the kingdom of England should be confirmed in the possession of the Duke;

3. He would place a garrison of the Duke's knights in the castle at Dover and maintain these at his own care and cost;

4. In other parts of England at the pleasure of the Duke he would maintain garrisons at other castles and make provision for their sustenance.

Harold would have to be out of his mind to have made such commitments. It is unbelievable that the premier earl of England, however disloyal he might be to his king, should have thus sworn away the kingdom – and his own future.

What does the Tapestry actually show in its pictures? It tells a vivid story indeed. Harold is seen receiving his orders from King Edward the Confessor; praying with his men for a safe journey at Bosham, on an inlet of Chichester Harbour, where he had a manor; embarking there with hawk and hound, shown prominently being carried aboard a waiting ship; being arrested by Guy, Count of Ponthieu, as soon as he sets foot on the coast of what is now northern France (NB : the Latin inscription woven into the Tapestry says that

he landed 'with the wind full in his sails', which may well be taken
to indicate that he was being blown off course by a gale).

Next, messengers from Duke William are seen demanding
Harold's release. Guy, who had once been William's prisoner and so
knew the man with whom he was dealing, complies. The Tapestry
goes on to show William paying Harold the rare compliment of
going out to meet and escort him from Eu, where William's lands
abutted upon Guy's, to the ducal palace of Rouen. There he
receives Harold in formal audience and then takes him as a fellow
warrior on a military foray during which Harold is shown dis-
tinguishing himself by gallantly rescuing two of William's soldiers
who have been caught in quicksands. For this and, one presumes,
also as a reward for good service during the expedition, Harold
is ceremonially given arms, or knighted, by William.

Now comes the crucial phase of the story. In one of the most
graphic panels of the Tapestry Harold is seen making a sacred
oath to William. He does so with arms outstretched so that each
hand rests lightly on holy relics, reported by William of Poitiers
to be the bones of saints. William sits on a throne and points mean-
ingly at Harold, as if to admonish him about the gravity of what
he is doing. Two people in attendance, one Norman and the other
English, are shown in similar postures. There is no doubt that the
meaning of all these gestures is to emphasize the solemnity of
Harold's commitment and consequently to magnify his later offence
in repudiating it. Many other such touches and implications add
to the impact of this segment of the Tapestry and betray its propagandist purpose. Thus, William's power as a ruler and his prowess as
a warrior are emphasized. Harold is similarly saluted – to add to
the glory of William in ultimately defeating him. William's supposed
knighting of Harold may well be interpreted as intended to impress
all military men with Harold's perfidy in 'usurping' the throne of
England and basely scorning his oath of allegiance to William.

The longer one studies the Tapestry the more do its deep purposes
become clear. So also does an impression that it might represent
a most skilful adaptation and extension of true facts. In this connection a curious circumstance may be mentioned which could have
much more bearing upon the tale told by the Tapestry than has
been recognized. Harold paid a visit to the continent of Europe in
the autumn of 1056. Proof of this is provided by a document, which
survives to this day, showing that he was among the witnesses and

signatories to a diploma issued at St Omer on 13 November by Baldwin the Fifth, Count of Flanders, a principality directly across the English Channel from Dover. The document is of little historical significance; it merely confirmed ownership by the Abbey of St Peter's at Ghent of their house at Harnes which was threatened with seizure by Count Eustace the Second of Boulogne. But the fact that it records the presence of 'Duke Harold' (the usual continental style of describing noble English titles is used) is of more than passing interest, since another signatory to the document is the same Guy of Ponthieu who, according to the Tapestry, captured Harold. This raises a possibility that Harold in fact made only one visit to Europe and went to St Omer not as Guy's captive but as his guest, and that the creators of the Tapestry conveniently altered dates and circumstances in concocting their story of Harold's visit to William, which quite probably never took place at all. A piece of evidence which strengthens doubt is that the Norman chroniclers and the Tapestry do not agree about the precise location of Harold's supposed visit to William. The Tapestry places the event at Bayeux, William of Poitiers at Bonneville, and Ordericus Vitalis (an Anglo-Norman scribe) at Rouen.

The Tapestry is now on permanent display in Bayeux, its original home and the ancient seat of the bishop who ordered its creation. Since the end of World War II its home has been an exhibition gallery on the first floor of the former Bishop's Palace in the lovely old town. It is exhibited behind glass at eye level round the walls of the room and is lit by a gentle light to prevent its colours from fading further. Not much is known about its history since it was finished, probably in 1077, but it is thought to have lain in obscurity in and near Bayeux for almost 700 years, until it was rediscovered by a Monsieur Lancelot, a French academician, in 1724. The Tapestry had miraculously survived fire, war, pillage and neglect during the intervening centuries but it had not survived intact. Some of its panels were frayed and damaged and, worse still, a concluding segment is believed to have disappeared entirely, perhaps rotted away or even wilfully destroyed. But by far the greater portion of the original work remains as a priceless memento of one of the most fateful events in medieval history and as a perpetual challenge to scholars and historians.

The Mystery of Aelfgyva

One charming but puzzling fact about the Tapestry is the inclusion
here and there of panels which seem to have no connection with
the principal theme. Perhaps they were placed there as a kind of
bait to attract the interest of simple folk who would not otherwise
view the Tapestry. Also, here and there the decorative panels
which adorn its top and bottom edges are diverted from their
portrayal of country activities such as ploughing, harrowing and
bird-scaring, sketches of legendary birds and animals, and the
illustration of fables, to revelatory side-aspects of the main story.
These include the stripping of the dead after the battle of Hastings
– even, apparently, during it – and, most surprisingly, certain
drawings which today would be classed as pornographic but in the
eleventh century might have been seen as providing bawdy light
relief. Nevertheless, it is difficult to explain the inclusion in the
upper border towards the end of the Tapestry of a naked man and
woman purposefully approaching each other, like amatory wrestlers,
above a main panel depicting William's army advancing to the
battlefield at Hastings. One is driven to some rather implausible
explanations. Could it possibly be that this little extravaganza is
meant to indicate that the English populace was so indifferent to
the attack upon Harold that it did not even interrupt its sexual
preoccupations while William's host was advancing to battle with
the alleged usurper?

In the case of one of these suggestive drawings, however, there
does seem to be a connection with the Tapestry's purpose, which
has so far gone undetected. The present author now offers it for
consideration. In a very narrow panel, placed between one of
ordinary dimensions showing Harold and William arriving at
William's palace and another illustrating their departure for the
military expedition discussed earlier, a fully-gowned woman is
seen apparently being caressed on the cheek by the outstretched
hand of a man striking a distinctive attitude, with the other hand
resting upon his hip. In the border immediately below the panel
is a naked man in exactly the same posture. A spectacular physical
attribute of this quaint exhibitionist is his enormous genitalia, shown
dangling grotesquely, and even impossibly, between his splayed
legs.

The legend in Latin on the mysterious main panel reads: *Ubi unus clericus et Aelfgyva* (Where a certain clergyman and Aelfgyva). No verb or other word clarifies the meaning of the panel, or helps to explain why the panel was included in the Tapestry at this point. Aelfgyva is, of course, a purely Anglo-Saxon name and the possibility immediately suggests itself that she went with Harold on his supposed visit to William's court. The man depicted with her is a clergyman or perhaps a monk, for his head is tonsured and he wears some form of clerical gown. Whether he is Norman or English is unclear. What does seem clear is that the way he is described – 'a certain clergyman' – is intended to convey that he was in some way notorious and that there was no need to mention his name because people knew who he was. The inference that he was mixed up in some scandal is strengthened by the lewd sub-panel.

The next question is : What can possibly be the association between the clothed pair and the naked man below them who is apeing the stance of the clergyman? Two possibilities offer themselves here. One rests on the assumption that Aelfgyva is not being caressed but is being reproached or even slapped by the clergyman for some sin, and the crude but highly effective drawing of the naked man below suggests that her sin was sexual. The other possibility is that Aelfgyva had had or was having an affair with a clergyman or monk and that the naked figure was introduced to denote the real interest of the clothed man in the panel whose attitude he is imitating so closely. The crudity of the lower picture is understandable when we remember that nine out of ten people viewing the Tapestry in the eleventh and twelfth centuries could not read – but they could certainly see. They would thoroughly enjoy the panel when the wording was explained to them. We can imagine them chuckling and saying, 'Oh oh, we know who *that* is.'

Whatever the explanation, it seems very likely that the intention was the same as that of the Tapestry as a whole – to strike at Harold – and if we cannot identify the clergyman we can perhaps do rather better in finding out who the woman might have been. Aelfgyva, spelt in a number of readily recognizable ways, was a common name in medieval England and occurs several times among the high-born women mentioned in the Anglo-Saxon Chronicle and in other records. One Aelgifu, the widow of King Edmund (941–946), was canonized. Another married King Edwig (955–959), a son of Edmund, but the marriage was dissolved by Archbishop Oda a year before Edwig died, on grounds of consanguinity. Yet another Aelgifu was the mistress or first wife of King Ethelred (976–1016), but as she died before 1002 she can scarcely be linked with the Tapestry. A fourth woman of the same name, Aelgifu of Northampton, was the mistress of the celebrated King Canute (1016–1035). She likewise lived a little too early to be confidently associated with the panel although there was certainly a scandalous rumour about her. It was said that her reputed son, later King Harold Harefoot (1037–1040), was not her son at all but a changeling, the child of a servant placed secretly in Aelgifu's bed to take the place of her own dead or stillborn baby in one of those pieces of skulduggery often suspected in English and other histories whenever noble or royal succession is at stake.

Only two likely candidates can compete for the distinction – or should it be the dishonour? – of being the woman in the panel. Unfortunately so little is known about one of them that there is even some doubt that she ever lived. She is Aelfgyva (or Alvive, another variant of the name), a supposed sister of Harold. Some scholars have claimed to have found a reference to her in the Domesday Book but even this is not certain. Some chroniclers asserted long after the Conquest that Harold pledged her in betrothal to a Norman noble as part of the bargain sealed during that much-debated visit he is said to have paid to William. Could it be that the panel shows her being led by the clergyman to the betrothal ceremony? It is faintly possible but hardly a convincing explanation of the drawings in the Tapestry.

The only other woman who could fit into the panel, is the Aelfgyva who in 1066 became Harold's mother-in-law, only a few months before he was killed at Hastings. She was the widow of Alfgar, Earl of Mercia. Again, little of substance is known about her except that she certainly came from spirited Anglo-Saxon stock. Her own mother-in-law was Lady Godiva, the heroine of the well-known legend of Peeping Tom. Perhaps Aelfgiva was even more venturesome than Godiva. We shall never know: The mystery of the woman and 'a certain clergyman' will endure.

To say that the Tapestry cannot be accepted as a true record of the Conquest is not to say, of course, that it is to be dismissed as worthless. In matters of detail such as clothing, armour, weapons, the kinds of boats used then and the ways they were built and sailed, its panels provide unique, convincing and marvellously revealing pictorial testimony. The portrayals in its early panels of hounds and hawks being taken aboard ship by Harold and his friends tell much about how sport was enjoyed in those days (besides causing some people to believe that any visit to northern Europe paid by Harold was purely an unofficial one to enjoy the chase in unfamiliar country and had nothing whatever to do with matters of State). Moreover, the Tapestry's vigorous version of William's subsequent invasion and victory, although so skilfully biassed, has furnished a basis upon which historians and other investigators have been able to build.

Much of the confusion and contradiction which swirls around the whole story would have been dissipated, if even the battlefield and the rest of the campaigning area of Sussex and Kent had yielded some tangible evidence. Unhappily, not one relic or fragment, not a vestige of bone or even a rusted piece of steel or other metal has emerged from the field of combat. This singular void has led to all manner of theorizing, from an extreme suggestion that the battle never happened to theories that it was fought elsewhere, or that it was a mere skirmish in which Duke William routed a small mob of ill-armed guerillas who were the only Anglo-Saxons to make any kind of resistance to him. Abundant evidence of savage hand-to-hand fighting at Senlac existed, presumably, for a considerable but unknown period after it ended, but everything had gone by the time, some decades later, that the paramount historical meaning of the battle had become clear and skilled investigators starting poking around the battlefield for anything they could find to fill in the picture. We may presume that clerks and others fitted by birth and brains to be classed above the unsparked peasantry would be looking for such evidence by 1100, when there could be no further doubt that during his turbulent and uneven reign lasting until 1087 King William had successfully imposed a new ruling house upon England and consequently that the battle of Hastings had inaugurated a new epoch. But the early searchings and all the others that have followed yielded nothing.

An explanation offered locally to account for the total lack of residual signs of the battle is that the ground upon which it was fought is sandy and porous. Geologists confirm that now, well over 900 years later, any surviving relics will have sunk many feet below surface level. But they are not beyond retrieval by modern methods and we can hope that one day a scientific effort will be made to reach some of them. There might not after all be very much to find, for the conflict, although savage, was of small scope in comparison with later massive battles in Europe, but even the smallest items found could tell us something exhilaratingly new. Nobody knows exactly how many soldiers fought at Hastings but the number could not possibly have been greater than 15,000 and was probably much smaller. Also, the fighting lasted only a few hours – perhaps six hours, allowing for inevitable pauses – and the weapons used were axes, swords, maces, javelins, bows and arrows, and even stones hurled from slings. Many would quickly perish, but surely some would still be there deep below the grass and topsoil. Looters would also have been at work as soon as any danger had passed; as we have noted, the Tapestry shows men stripping armour and vestments off fallen warriors even before the fighting was over. The thieves and pillagers, concerned only with plunder, would have had no inkling of the historic importance of what had happened that Saturday in October 1066. They behaved like the robbers who looted the tombs of the Pharaohs in Egypt two and three thousand years earlier. But they would not have taken *everything* away from the field. It seems inconceivable that no historical treasure of any kind lies deep but retrievable.

Such evidence as is available today, including the Tapestry, leaves little doubt that a fearful clash did take place on the meadow known as Senlac which one can still inspect from the ruins of Battle Abbey, or from a country road skirting its low-lying southern boundary. The Battle of Hastings, however, remains an enigma. It poses a score of questions which have aroused but exasperated historians and scholars for nearly 1,000 years. Here are just a few of them. Was Harold fighting in a just cause on behalf of his kingdom, or was he an unscrupulous throne-grabber who could command no national following? Why did he race down the length of England to offer William battle precipitately and with a tired and battered army? What role did Edith Swan Neck play in his life and fate? What influence did the other high-born women have upon events on both sides of the English Channel before the Conquest? Did William have a valid claim to the throne of England? What were the vital factors that made him choose Pevensey and the area of Hastings for his invasion? Were others in collusion with him in 1066? Was Harold a murderer, like his father?

To some such questions answers will here be offered; to some there will never be answers.

2

Noble Triangle:
Duke, King and Earl

Let us now set the stage for our story by considering the contrasting personalities of the two principals who were destined to face each other at Hastings in a winner-take-all struggle for one of the choicest kingdoms in the known world of their time. Neither had a natural right of succession to that kingdom, and there were others who brooded and schemed to seize it for themselves. But these two men dwarfed the rest – the first, Harold, because he was the man in possession and the second, William, because he had the material means and the determination, thoroughness and audacity to undertake one of the most daring gambles Europe had yet seen. He would face far more formidable odds than the trail-blazing but purely colonizing expedition made by Julius Caesar against the unlettered and ill-equipped natives of the same island more than 1,000 years earlier.

There is no doubt that, of the two, William was the more forceful, the more cunning schemer and the more effective leader. He needed these advantages to have any chance of overcoming the great geographic and military odds against him. As befitted an ambitious aggressor, William was a big man physically as well as mentally. The surviving drawings and pictures show him as tall and conspicuously broad-shouldered. He was 38 years old when he set out to conquer England, just beginning to lose that youthful trimness which had graced him during half a lifetime spent contending with the challenges and rigours of eleventh-century existence. He had an air of dignity and authority appropriate to one who had had to plot and fight for survival from childhood on. His dark, receding hair served as much to enhance his aura of command as to denote the passage of youth. His neck was shaven high at the back in the fashion of the Norman nobility, and he sported two thin, twirling moustaches on a firm and stubborn-looking upper lip.

In character, his two most prominent traits were his coolness and his shrewdness. They combined to make him cautious and calculating, not given to excesses of either mind or body. 'If his voice was harsh, what he said was always suited to the occasion,' wrote an anonymous Norman monk whose simple obituary of him has survived. The quality of self-defence had been developed in William from his very birth. He had to overcome the stigma of illegitimacy which, even though it meant far less in those uninhibited days than later, was still a damaging mark against one who on his father's side was in a position to contend for power within the ruling class of Normandy but on his mother's could hardly have been of more lowly status. He was the natural son of a feudal overlord, Robert the Devil, Duke of Normandy, and Arletta, the daughter of Fulbert, a peasant who was primarily a tanner but also a jack-of-several-trades, including those of embalmer and tailor. (Arletta was born and bred in Falaise, a settlement 19 miles from Caen from which just under nine centuries later, an invading force containing many soldiers with Norman and English blood in their veins burst out to pursue and eventually crush an enemy hailing from beyond the Rhine, the wide river which had been, even long before Arletta's time, a barrier between East and West Europe.)

Duke Robert first noticed Arletta as he was riding on horseback through Falaise. One story of their encounter says that he saw her dancing at the roadside and stopped to speak to her. Another has it that he saw her as she was washing clothes at a roadside stream. She surely captivated Duke Robert, and to do so she must have been more than usually attractive, as she strolled among the few simple huts of wattle and daub, and an occasional one of rough stone, which made up the Falaise of her day. She has a twofold claim to attention as a human factor in medieval history. She was the mother not only of William the Conqueror but of another boy born some nine years later who was to serve as William's right-hand man almost to the end of their lifetimes. This was the formidable Odo of Bayeux. He was a legitimate son of Arletta by Herluin de Conte-ville, who married her (perhaps under duress) after the powerful Duke Robert had finished with her. She thus became the Viscountess de Conteville, a grand title for the former peasant girl who had happened to catch the eye of her feudal lord and master. She was an early example of the low-born courtesan who contributed importantly to the genealogical tables of the nobility as well as to the history books. Arletta's family climbed the social scale with her. Fulbert the Tanner, her father, became a supervising attendant of the noble bedchamber of Conteville. Arletta's brothers, Osbern and Walter, were given jobs at their sister's court.

Arletta had had another illegitimate child, a daughter, some time before she married de Conteville. The girl, who was named Adelaide, may have been another product of the liaison between Arletta and Duke Robert. Adelaide made almost as distinguished a show as her mother, and certainly a more respectable one. She made three marriages of quality – to Enguerrand Count of Ponthieu, to Lambert of Lens, and finally to Odo, Count of Champagne. Arletta's life was full, but short. She is believed to have died in 1050, about 40 years old.

William made good use of his younger brother Odo. Some ten years before he invaded England, while he was still securing his hold upon his duchy, he needed a reliable ecclesiastical prop to his temporal authority. He appointed Odo as Bishop of Bayeux at the remarkably early age of 19, long before Odo could possibly have gained the spiritual knowledge appropriate to the high office. It was a calculating and cynical appointment, typical of the ambitious and unscrupulous William. Anybody less suitable than Odo for the post would have been hard to find. The evidence shows that he was all that William was not. He was coarse, lustful, brutal and greedy and consequently a far more typical figure of his era than the unusually prim William, whose inclinations directed him much more powerfully towards exercise of the mind than gratification of the body. Odo fought at William's side at Hastings, using a studded mace to club men to death instead of gashing them with a sword. It is said against him that he could thereby make the grim pretence that, as he smote his enemies, he was not disobeying an edict of the church of Rome that its servants should not spill blood.

These two men of deeply contrasting characters complemented each other, and for 16 years after the Conquest Odo served William well as his administrative deputy. But his base nature finally betrayed him. Five years before William died he had Odo summarily arrested in the Isle of Wight. The nature of Odo's crime is not known, but we can assume that it was probably some form of treason, perhaps even a move to dethrone the ageing William, for William formally deprived Odo of his earldom of Kent, despatched him to prison in Normandy, and seemed resolved to keep him there permanently. Only as he felt death approaching in 1087 did he unwillingly agree to the appeals of those around him to set Odo free. 'There is no doubt that if he is released he will disturb the whole country and be the ruin of thousands,' William is quoted as saying. The dismal prophecy was soon fulfilled. Within one year of William's death Odo was leading a plot against the throne and was despoiling many areas of the country. His machinations failed and at the end of 1088 he left England and never returned.

William was only eight years old when he succeeded his father, who died suddenly at Nicaea (now in Turkey) while returning home from a pilgrimage of repentance to Jerusalem. It proved barely possible for a long time to keep the boy on the ducal throne. Plot after plot was made against his life and some of his guardians lost their lives in defending him. Among these unfortunates was one of Arletta's brothers, Osbern, who was killed during a scuffle in the boy's bedroom while kidnappers were trying to make off with William and destroy him. It is a pity that so little is known of the story of William's turbulent boyhood, for it would have made a classic among history's true melodramas. The lives and fortunes of his loyal relatives and supporters depended upon his survival and they often had to keep him hidden for weeks at a time to protect him from other relatives and would-be usurpers. Arletta's other brother, Walter, was one who preserved him. It is recorded that he often awakened the boy in the middle of the night and hastened off with him to some lowly and inconspicuous hiding place in Bayeux.

William's vulnerability in these early years was the greater, of course, because of his illegitimacy. It seriously weakened his hold upon the succession and gave his enemies a useful battle-cry against him; their sneering description of him as 'William the Bastard' was to haunt him all his life, as also was the humble origin of his mother's family. The duchy on which in these first years he and his supporters kept precarious hold was by no means stable. It had been founded only a century and a half earlier (compare this with the 500 years of authenticated royalty in England) by Danish Viking bands. They had been repulsed in their colonizing onslaughts against England by King Alfred the Great and, turning southwards, had eventually surged into northern Europe.

Normandy had been born when the Danish leader, Rollo, decided to settle in the lower basin of the river Seine and was joined there by other Vikings who liked the look of the fertile, well-watered coastal terrain. Rollo and his followers softened somewhat as their stake in the land grew. They turned to Christianity, embracing this new faith with the same extreme ardour with which they had earlier perpetrated their bloodthirsty missions of plunder and rapine. Like that other strong race, the Romans, they had the knack of absorbing peoples and cultures. By the time William was born they had abandoned their Norse tongue for Latin and a musical native language called Romance, the forerunner of modern French, and built themselves up into one of the most progressive new races in Europe. Their church was strong, their aristocracy proud and brave. But this did not mean that they had lost the fire of their Viking inheritance. They were still tough, stubborn, energetic and aggressive – and they loved fighting and combat almost as fiercely as their ancestors; so much so indeed that when there was no war to be fought, no neighbour to be chased off their territory, and no palace feud or revolution to be prosecuted, they spent their energies in mock combat among themselves.

It is not surprising that there were many challengers for William's throne, among them some valid claims for the right to replace him on account of his illegitimacy. His paternal grandfather (Duke Richard the Third) had had six legitimate children, all of whose descendants could claim that their link with the throne was at least purer that William's, even if it were not quite so close, and many of whom were ready to fight their elder rivals in the brood as well as William for a chance to govern the thriving duchy. The English historian, Professor David C. Douglas, who has made a close study of William and his times, asserts that the period of his minority after 1037 was one of the darkest periods in Norman history. Lawlessness and local feudal fighting was so widespread that villagers formed themselves into armed bands to defend themselves and their property, often under the command of their village priest.

But as William grew up and showed himself even in early youth to be not only a capable warrior in the Viking mould but an individual with unusually promising qualities of firmness and leadership, the challenges and rebellions against him steadily diminished. His most powerful ally in crushing them was King Henry I of

France, his neighbour to the south-east and his overlord under an arrangement made many years earlier by his ducal grandfather in the days when Normandy had been a weak, fledgling nation. King Henry had formally recognized William, even though a child, as the lawful Duke of Normandy in 1035 and thereafter had exercised his military and political power towards keeping William alive and *in situ*. It was greatly to his advantage to do so. By maintaining William he also maintained his own sovereignty over Normandy, which would be renounced by a usurper, and at the same time he was putting William into his debt at an early and impressionable age.

It was Henry who eventually preserved William at the age of 18 from the last and most dangerous challenge of all and, in doing so, decisively influenced the destiny not only of Normandy but also of England. If William had been ousted and killed a new dynasty would have been installed in Normandy and the conquest of England might never have been attempted. The man who raised this last rebellion in his own interest was Count Guy of Burgundy, a cousin of William and one of the legitimate grandchildren of the Duke Richard mentioned above. He persuaded a considerable company of other Norman magnates to join him in a determined plot to get rid of William so that Guy could become duke and share out the duchy with them. The conspirators' first move was to try to kill William in an ambush at Valognes, 15 miles south east of Cherbourg. Some spy or defector warned William of his danger and the young duke fled by night across country to his home at Falaise. There he learned of the magnitude of the plot against him and realized that without help he could not hope to defeat it. Leaving some of his sparse forces to hamper and delay Guy's army, which was now deployed in north-west Normandy and was advancing upon Falaise, William rode off to seek intervention on his behalf by Henry, his overlord. They met at Poissy, 15 miles west of Paris, and Henry promptly raised an army to support his young vassal. He led it across the frontier into Normandy to confront the rebels, joined on the way by William's smaller force which had made a sortie from Falaise with the rebels advancing behind it. The encounter came at Val-es-Dunes, in the heart of territory which was to be fought over once again in World War II, nine centuries later.

Surviving accounts of the battle are confusing and downright contradictory in many details. The one point upon which they agree is that Guy and his fellow rebels were thoroughly beaten, several hundreds of men being pushed back into the river and drowned. The most distorted versions of the battle are supplied by William's scribes and chroniclers. They exaggerate his role in the fighting to make him figure as a superlative warrior and they carefully falsify his relationship with Henry. They were writing many years later when William's conquering role in history had been established, and they naturally did not wish to emphasize that at any time in his career was he a vassal who, in extremity, had had to beg for the help of his overlord. So their versions of the battle of Val-es-Dunes give the impression that William and Henry were fighting side by side as equals and that, if anything, victory was due more to the prowess of William than to the leadership of the older and more experienced King Henry. Such distortions serve to strengthen suspicions about the validity of the events leading to the Conquest as reported in the Bayeux Tapestry, for if Norman chroniclers could produce twisted accounts of the suppression of the revolt of Guy of Burgundy, they could well do the same with Harold of England's visit to William's court and even the Battle of Hastings itself.

William's hold upon Normandy was never again seriously challenged, and his victory over Guy brought other extraordinary but valuable consequences. A few months after the battle, in October 1047, an ecclesiastical council was convened by William at Caen, at which an innovation called The Truce of God was proclaimed. This remarkable ordinance prohibited private warfare every week from Wednesday night until Monday morning, cramming the prosecution of feuds and other opportunities for blood-letting into the first part of the week; it also banned private fighting altogether during such holy seasons as Advent, Lent, Easter and Pentecost, under penalty of excommunication. Only King Henry and Duke William were exempted from observing the Truce and were required to maintain armies at readiness to go into the field at any time in the public interest, in their domains and as allies.

Everybody swore on holy relics to observe the Truce of God, but the persistence of uprisings against William, on a diminishing scale, until about 1054 – seven years during which he was tightening his grip on his domain – suggests that the observance was neither generally kept nor strictly enforced. But it is a revealing measure.

It implies firstly that private warfare in Normandy in the middle of the eleventh century was about as normal an element of existence as animal hunting. It also shows that the Church pragmatically recognized its inability to eradicate strife and aggression and limited itself to trying to curb them. We may be tempted to feel lofty amusement at such a Truce but we should pause to ask ourselves whether ordering men to lay aside their arms between sunset on Wednesday and dawn on Monday is so very much less enlightened than arranging for armies of the twentieth century to observe an armistice during the lunar New Year in Vietnam, in an undeclared war many thousands of miles away from the homeland of at least one of the contestants.

It is scarcely surprising, considering that William was continually fighting off domestic insubordination and foreign assaults upon his authority until he was approaching 30 years of age, that he should have matured quickly as a resourceful, cunning and ruthless ruler and warrior. It was also inevitable, as his military and political stature grew, that he should find his relationship with his overlord Henry of France, irksome. The final break between them in 1052 signalled the collapse of the Truce of God which they were supposed jointly to maintain. Two years after their quarrel, Henry joined other foreigners in an invasion of Normandy which William squashed, thereby putting a permanent stop to Henry's machinations against him.

There is abundant evidence that William knew the efficacy of short but sharp ferocity in asserting his will over men who opposed him militarily or politically or sought otherwise to thwart him. He demonstrated this early in his career as a soldier and confirmed it many times after he had conquered England. Once, during his middle twenties, he made a surprise attack under cover of darkness upon rebels who had gathered to resist him in a fortress at Alençon, on the southern fringe of his duchy. As he approached the town some of the people taunted him, it is said, by thumping upon hides and shouting 'Tanner! Tanner! The bastard tanner is here!' The cries died away as William stormed the town, but he did not forget them. In full view of the men defending the inner castle he had the hands and feet of his tormentors hacked off. The effect was immediate. His awed opponents lost their stomach for resisting him further in their citadel. They surrendered; and news of what had happened at Alençon spread to another town, Domfront, some

40 miles away, which had also been rising against him. Domfront gave up the fight in return for William's promise of mercy.

Even while he was still establishing himself in his own duchy William was already looking speculatively across the Channel. He was on most friendly terms with Edward the Confessor, the venerable reigning monarch of England, who had passed most of his early life in Normandy. In about 1051 William astutely used this friendship as a basis for his concocted claim upon the throne of England. One important point to emphasize in estimating the validity or otherwise of William's claim is that it was based solely on statements by William himself and by his Norman mouthpieces. It was never confirmed in any legal or other official document which has survived in either Normandy or England. Sometimes even William's own native biographers have difficulty in confirming it. One of them let the cat out of the bag, inadvertently or perhaps by design in the interests of historical truth, many years later. The admission that William's claim was spurious is made twice in one of the most remarkable documents of the period, the *Ecclesiastical History* written by Ordericus Vitalis, a monk who grew up during William's lifetime and who spent most of his own life in an abbey in Normandy. In this History, written in the first half of the twelfth century, Ordericus Vitalis gives a highly detailed account of the life and death of William. In describing William's last hours he uses a device originated by Thucydides, the peerless Greek historian, 15 centuries earlier. Vitalis allows the subject to tell his own story in the form of an address or confession to those about him as he prepares himself for death. He causes William to say: 'I have placed on my brow a royal diadem, which none of my predecessors wore, having acquired it by the grace of God, not by hereditary right.' Then, half a dozen paragraphs later, he has William repeating this illuminating admission in different and far more damning words: 'I appoint no one my heir to the crown of England but leave it to the disposal of the eternal Creator, whose I am, and who ordereth all things. For I did not attain that high honour by hereditary right, but wrested it from the perjured King Harold in a desperate battle, with much effusion of human blood, and it was by the slaughter and banishment of his adherents that I subjected England to my rule.'

Notwithstanding the highly unusual manner in which Ordericus Vitalis tells his story, these passages carry a good deal of conviction, particularly since the writer is demonstrably accurate in the rest of his History. It should also be borne in mind that by putting the words into William's mouth so ingeniously he avoids the distasteful responsibility of serving truth by directly branding his king as a usurper. Ordericus Vitalis is by no means a witness hostile to William; a reading of his work seems to show that he was an honest and devout man who set himself the task of recording facts as justly and as fully as he could. His History compares well with that of William of Poitiers, whose *The Deeds of William, Duke of the Normans and King of the English* is marked by slippery verbiage and shaky genealogy and is as demonstrably inaccurate as that of Ordericus Vitalis is sound. On the topic of William's right to the throne of England, Poitiers says : 'This land he gained as the legal heir with the confirmation of the oaths of the English. He took possession of his inheritance by battle, and he was crowned at last with the consent of the English, or at least with the desire of their magnates. And if it be asked what was his hereditary title, let it be answered that a close kinship existed between King Edward and the son of Duke Robert (i.e. William) whose paternal aunt, Emma, was the sister of Duke Richard the Third and the mother of King Edward himself.'

It would be tedious to go into the ramifications of the relationships quoted so smoothly by William of Poitiers. Suffice it to say that they confirm Duke William's claim to the throne of Normandy (provided his illegitimacy is overlooked) but they place him no nearer to the throne of England than several other distant kinsmen and descendants of King Canute (1016–1035) and Ethelred (979–1016). Truth to tell, he had no serious hereditary claim at all. He was in fact William the Conqueror.

A Year of Commotion

William cloaked his naked aggression with the story, already noted, that in 1051 Edward had promised him the throne of England when the time came. The Worcester edition of the Anglo-Saxon Chronicle records that William came to England in that year but says nothing about his purpose or that during his stay Edward promised him anything at all. It states : 'Then soon came Duke William from

B

beyond the sea with a great retinue of Frenchmen, and the King received him with as many of his companions as it pleased him, and let him go again.' This is a quite definite record of a visit, although the references to the limitation upon the number of Frenchmen whom King Edward would receive and 'let him go again' are quaint, and any hidden meanings they might have cannot now be satisfactorily divined. Some historians claim that the visit never happened, dismissing the reference to it with the rather over-confident assertion that the monk at Worcester simply got his facts wrong. They say (a) that William was so involved in the turbulent affairs of his duchy that year that he could not have afforded the risk of being absent from it for as long as a visit to England would have demanded, and (b) that none of the other chroniclers mentions the visit in their entries for the year. The first contention has some merit but it is not conclusive, and the second can be met with an explanation that so much happened during the year 1051 in England that the chroniclers were hard pressed to include everything in their writings. It was one of the most momentous and exciting years in the immediate pre-Conquest period in England and if, as seems likely, William did use it for a trip, even a comparatively brief one in the later months of the year, to sue for a promise of the succession, he could not have chosen a moment better suited to his purpose. It seems indeed to have been a moment which demanded a political sortie by him, no matter what were his preoccupations at home and the risks he took in being away from Normandy. England had been in turmoil and very close to civil war at the end of the summer, and now William's most powerful adversaries in the country, members of a family dedicated to preserving it from foreign influences and incursions because they wanted the succession to the throne for themselves, were temporarily in eclipse. King Edward, William's friend, had managed to win a bloodless victory over them and was in firmer control of England than he had ever been or was to be again. He had ousted Earl Godwin, who for some years had been virtually running the country for him, as well as his five sons – including Harold, who was destined to fulfil the family hopes for the throne 15 years later but only briefly and catastrophically. In a trial of strength with the Godwin clan Edward had had the eager support of other earls who were only too pleased to be offered a chance of toppling their over-powerful rival.

Godwin and his family had been banished, ostensibly because

they had refused to obey an order by Edward to punish the inhabitants of Dover for having attacked a party of Normans led by Count
Eustace of Boulogne (the husband of Goda, Edward's sister) while
they were going home across the Channel from a visit to Edward's
court. The chronicles of the year are ample in their accounts of
a bloody brawl between Eustace's men and the Dover townspeople
and its consequences. Their accounts vary in detail and emphasis
according to the writers' antipathies to the flock of Norman
courtiers which Edward was gathering at his court, but the basic
facts are clear enough. Eustace and his party autocratically demanded lodgings overnight in Dover and they attacked and killed
one householder who refused. A fight of considerable ferocity then
developed between foreigners and townspeople. Eustace and his
surviving companions, who do not seem to have fared too well in the
fighting, rode off to complain to Edward about what had happened.
Edward listened and without waiting to hear the other side's
account ordered Godwin to punish the Englishmen. It was too much
for Godwin to stomach. He refused to carry out the order for various
reasons; he disbelieved Eustace's one-sided account, the people of
Dover were inhabitants of Godwin's earldom and his own folk,
and Edward's favouritism towards his Norman friends and courtiers
was becoming obnoxious.

However, the incident seems hardly important enough to explain
the explosion which followed, and it most probably happened at
just the right moment to bring to a head a dispute which had been
simmering for a long time between the king, a weak but petulant
ruler, and his ambitious chief lieutenant. The clue to this is to be
found in the Chronicles. Several writers infuse their annals with
oblique but unmistakable references to the resentment felt by many
Englishmen at Edward's almost obsessive favouritism of his Norman
friends. One goes into long detail about the appointment by Edward
of a Norman, Robert of Jumièges, to the supreme ecclesiastical post
of Archbishop of Canterbury and the prompt refusal of the new
archbishop to confirm the appointment of an English abbot (whose
name Sparhafoc, meaning Sparrowhawk, sounds comical to modern
ears) as Bishop of London. Another relates that 'the foreigners' had
built a castle in Herefordshire, in the territory of Godwin's eldest
son Sweyn, and 'inflicted all the injuries and insults they possibly
could upon the king's men in that region.'

So it is apparent that there was much more at issue between

the King and Godwin, supported by his family and his followers, than the incident at Dover. There is evidence in the records of Godwin's family of an angry quarrel between it and Archbishop Robert, who accused Godwin of having stolen lands belonging to the church and told tales to the king of other alleged wickednesses on the part of the man whom he hated and feared. Egged on by Robert, the king tried to impose his will upon Godwin but failed and eventually called a national council for 7 September to consider Godwin's insubordination. Everybody of importance in the country, from the king downwards, brought his army to the area. When Godwin and his sons placed their forces in a strong strategic position across the main track between Bristol and Oxford at Beverstone, 15 miles south of Gloucester, all the other earls in the kingdom summoned reinforcements to protect the king and at the same time to put down Godwin, of whom they were of course jealous. After a number of confrontations which developed almost to the point of bloodshed, Godwin realized that the odds against his overthrowing the king were too great, and he yielded – temporarily – to the royal justice. With so much force backing him, the King felt himself strong enough to allot Godwin and his family five days in which to leave the country. They obeyed. Godwin and three of his sons (Sweyn, Tostig and Gyrth) sailed across the Channel from Bosham to Flanders to accept shelter offered them by Count Baldwin, a relative by marriage. Harold and a younger brother, Leofwin, sailed from Bristol to Ireland, where there was still a thriving colony of Vikings and where King Diormid, a friend of Harold, received them at his castle in the growing city of Dublin.

King Edward had won a welcome liberation from years of domination by Godwin, and he made the most of it. He was inordinately vindictive in his triumph. His behaviour points to some remarkable frailties and deviations in his character which many analysts of him during succeeding centuries do not seem to have taken sufficiently into account. He included even his own wife, Edith, a daughter of Godwin, in the dismissal of the family from his home and court. It was an extraordinarily spiteful thing to do, for there is no evidence that she was in any way associated with the events leading to the outlawry. It sheds light not only on the nature of their relationship but on Edward's attitude towards women as a whole. It brought him discreetly-worded but none the less pointed reproof from the chroniclers: 'And soon after this [the banishment of Godwin] happened, the King forsook the Lady who had been consecrated his queen and he had her deprived of all that she owned in land and in gold and silver, and of everything and committed her to his sister, the abbess of Wherwell, near Winchester.' We may note that he did not do this to Edith in the heady moment of his triumph over Godwin but afterwards, deliberately and with thorough malice.

Royal Anti-Feminist

It was not the first time that Edward had behaved viciously to a woman close to him. It conformed to a pattern of anti-feminism which marked his life as king. For example, when in 1042 he succeeded his half-brother Harthacunute, he turned violently against his mother, Emma, the daughter of a Duke of Normandy. The episode is duly recorded in the Chronicle: 'Soon after, the King had all the lands which his mother owned confiscated for his own use and took from her all she possessed, an indescribable number of things of gold and silver, because she had been too tight-fisted with him.' There is no doubt that the maternal parsimony was by no means the only reason why Edward behaved thus and it is regarded as certain that Godwin, then marching towards his paramount position of authority in the land, jogged the insecure king into moving against her. Emma and Godwin hated each other. Six years earlier, in a fierce dispute over the succession to the throne caused by the awkward fact that King Canute had had sons both by Emma and his mistress (Aelgifu of Northampton), Godwin had sided with Emma's rivals and when she lost he had underlined her defeat by forcing her to leave England and take refuge in Flanders. This humiliation had followed an unsavoury event a year earlier when one of Emma's sons (Alfred) by her first marriage to King Ethelred had been murdered while travelling from Flanders to Winchester to see his mother. Emma along with many others had no doubt that Godwin was responsible for the murder, directly or otherwise, because he wanted Alfred out of the way to the throne, which he had reserved for his pliant tool, Edward.

Godwin's guilt must have been very obvious, for the usually

circumspect chroniclers did not hesitate to brand him. They even published a ballad about the crime which he had commissioned :

But then Godwin prevented him, and placed him in captivity,
Dispersing his followers besides, slaying some in various ways;
Some of them were sold for money, some cruelly murdered,
Some were put in chains, and some were blinded,
Some were mutilated, and some were scalped.
No more horrible deed was done in this land
After the Danes came and made peace with us here.
We can now but trust to the dear God
That they who were so pitiably killed
Rejoice joyfully in the presence of Christ.

Threatened with every kind of injury, the prince still lived
Until the decision was taken to convey him
To the city of Ely, in chains as he was.
As soon as he arrived, his eyes were put out on board ship
And thus sightless he was brought to the monks.
And there he remained as long as he lived.
Thereafter he was buried, as well became his rank,
With great ceremony, so honourable was he,
At the west end of the church, very near to the tower
In the south aisle. His soul is with Christ.

This ghastly episode reflects not only Godwin's character but the times in which he flourished so mightily. He had the necessary, if repellant, traits which ensured the grabbing of power in Saxon England and indeed in all parts of the known world in the eleventh century. He was determined to the extreme of utter ruthlessness, sweeping aside anything or anybody standing in his path, and so thinly civilized as to be still half-savage. As we follow the course of events leading to the field of Hastings, we should keep in mind the primitive standards of the era, rejecting the gilded pictures painted by latter-day novelists and romantics and accepting the principal players – William, Harold Godwinson, Harald Hardrada and Tostig – for what they really were.

Edward's attitude towards women is worth serious examination because it had such profound effects upon history. According to ample evidence, he either feared or disliked women and throughout his life wanted to have as little to do with them as he could. After he had married Edith, Godwin's daughter, he shunned her. The most revealing of his actions – or lack of them – towards her was his refusal to give her a child and his country an heir to the throne who might well have averted the Conquest had he succeeded Edward. This failure to produce an heir was incalculably important. It swayed the course of world history. If Edward and Edith had had a son soon after they were married in 1045, he would have been about 20 when Edward died in 1066. He would have been mature and there would probably have been little question of his succession. So Harold would never have sat upon the throne and William would have had no valid grounds for invading England because he could not possibly have challenged the heir, who would have been part-Norman himself. It is unlikely that even if William had wished to seize England he would have been able to gather enough support for an unprovoked and unjustified aggression. There would therefore have been no Norman Conquest. England's story would have been dramatically different and her influence upon the rest of the world would have been similarly altered. How different the world of today would be is quite impossible to imagine.

Some historians have inferred that Edward refused to have children because he felt himself to be more of a celibate priest and anointed king than an ordinary lusty man. The truth may be less lofty, deriving from physical instead of spiritual causes. We have implicit evidence that he did not have sexual relations with Edith. There is no evidence or suggestion that he ever had any such relations with other women, let alone that he ever begat illegitimate offspring in an age when this was a more or less usual practice. Lifelong sexual abstinence by Edward, for whatever reason, is in fact unequivocally proclaimed in a biography of him (and the House of Godwin), much of which is believed to have been written while he still lived. In *Vita Aedwardi Regis*, produced by an unknown author who was probably commissioned by Queen Edith to write what amounts to a eulogy of the royal family, it is said: 'He preserved the dignity of his consecration with holy chastity and lived his whole life dedicated to God in holy innocence.' The author also makes a striking statement which seems intended to indicate that Edith's role in Edward's life was not that of wife but of daughter. He quotes Edward as saying on his deathbed: 'She has served me devotedly and has always stood close by my side like a beloved daughter.' Surely this was about as far as a man actually commissioned and authorized by Edith herself could go in pointing to a secret of the marriage bed.

Another biographer writing 70 years after Edward's death went much further and is admittedly not to be taken too literally. He was Osbert of Clare, a monk of Suffolk who became Prior of Westminster and was devoted to promoting Edward's saintly aspect: He wrote: 'This young woman [Edith was almost half the age of Edward at the time, being scarcely more than 21 to his 40] was delivered to the royal bridal apartments with ceremonial rejoicing. . . . But merciful God, who preserved his blessed confessor Alexius a virgin, kept, as we believe, St Edward the King all the days of his life in the purity of the flesh. The excellent queen served him as a daughter. . . . But she preserved the secret of the king's chastity of which she had learned, and kept those counsels which she knew.'

Some modern scholars, notably Frank Barlow, Professor of History at Exeter University, who has contributed much to an understanding of Edward's life and times, doubt that Edward was sexually incapable towards woman or deliberately kept himself virginal. Professor Barlow quotes the above two passages in his copious biography of Edward and then rejects them sternly 'Not only is the story of Edward's virginity without good authority, it is also implausible, and, far from helping us to understand the situation and events, merely obscures. It is a typical example of that irrationality and ignorant credulity with which the eleventh century abounds.'

There is scope for such a judgement, but it cannot be allowed to go unchallenged. Is not 'good authority' provided by a biographer writing at the behest of and presumably with the approval of Edith herself? Why is the story of Edward's virginity implausible? Why should he not have been impotent? Many men have remained virgins all their lives, and many more have been impotent or homosexual. There can be no doubt that Edward's incapacity with women was widely believed in medieval times. Writing some 60 years after his death and presumably using statements from contemporaries and also possibly from writings which have since been lost, William of Malmesbury, a devout if flowery scribe, describes in lavish detail the relationship between Edward and Edith. He says in his history of the King of England:

Shortly after [in 1045] the King took Edgitha, the daughter of Godwin, to wife; a woman whose bosom was the school of every liberal art, though little skilled in earthly matters; on seeing her,

if you were amazed by her erudition, you must absolutely languish
for the purity of her mind and the beauty of her person. Both in
her husband's lifetime, and afterwards, she was not entirely
free from suspicion of dishonour; but when dying in the time of
King William, she voluntarily satisfied the bystanders of her
unimpaired chastity, by an oath. When she became his wife, the
King so artfully managed that he neither removed her from his
bed, nor knew her after the manner of men. I have not been able
to discover whether he acted thus from dislike of her family,
or out of pure regard to chastity; yet it is most notoriously affirmed
that he never violated his purity by connection with any woman.

The theme of Edward's purity was revived, spuriously, by clerics
sponsoring his proposed elevation to the sainthood. They told the
Pope in 1160 that when his tomb was opened in 1102, almost 40
years after he had died, his body was found to be soft and aromatic
and free of all corruption. In a prime exercise of medieval propaganda, they claimed that this was proof of his physical virginity,
and were apparently believed. We must concede that this is an
example of the 'irrationality and ignorant credulity' specified by
Professor Barlow. It adds nothing helpful for or against the case
regarding Edward's manhood.

On a practical level, a few other effective questions may be
asked about Edward. Was his extraordinary liking for the company
of virile Normans about him, taken in conjunction with his shunning
of women, a sign of latent, suppressed femininity within him? Was
the outward aspect of scholarly and monk-like asceticism which he
showed publicly a mask to hide his inner fears and knowledge
about himself and and his sexual inadequacies? If answers to such
questions were possible they would settle once and for all the
controversy about the true identity of Edward the so-called Confessor.

The topic of Edward's masculinity, or lack of it, is being studied
in the twentieth century with more precision than ever before as
analysis of sexual matters becomes increasingly scientific and frank,
especially in the United States. An illuminating contribution based
upon a study of existing evidence about Edward comes from
Joseph Oelbaum, the New York psychoanalytic-therapist, who
specialized for many years in treating patients whose problems
were founded upon sexual complications. His report on Edward
(made to the author in 1973) is as follows :

Apparently Edward's statements about his celibacy and his wife's affirmation of this satisfies nobody. More distant onlookers, in the main, have suggested that he was only impotent with his wife and not with other women—that he was impotent with women but not with men. Possibly celibacy in a king is regarded as unkingly. Divine Right notwithstanding, the psychoanalytic investigation of an individual remains essentially the same for king and mortal alike. . . . While societies and social structures have changed markedly; while child-rearing practices have undergone vast changes; though our subject be 900 years in the past, those things and inter-actions that developed humans then do so now; while the external world is now completely different from what it was then, the dynamics for growth and personality development, and with it health and mental disorder, remain essentially the same.

Regarding Edward's sexual milieu the facts that present themselves are his being childless, both he and his wife attesting to his celibacy, and – this tangentially – that homosexuality was quite the fashion among Royalty. With all this, with all the assertions and counter-assertions, and granted our need to have a 'functioning' king, the evidence does point to Edward being a true sexual celibate.

Edward's father, Ethelred, has been characterized as a weak and ineffectual man; on a simplistic level this picture would easily fit into a prime stereotype of the homosexual's male parent. Edward was abandoned, however figuratively, by this man and forced into exile with his mother. This alone would seem to present abundantly fertile ground for a great attachment to her, with a subsequent feminine identification for himself. This *might* have been were it not for Emma herself.

She is pictured as being parsimonious, miserly, withholding. (On a parent-child level this does not refer to material things alone but more likely than not typifies a general attitude, a level of feeling and affection that exists from parent towards child.) Unfortunately for one of the theories, as well as for Edward, she does not conform to the usual description of the homosexual's mother. That mother is usually quite seductive and 'loving' towards her male offspring – seemingly to substitute him for her ineffectual husband – overtly generous and giving, though covertly quite emasculating. Mother and son are known to form strong 'girlish' attachments to each other, she recognizing and supporting – forming – his 'feminity' by treating him as if he were one of the girls, by taking him shopping for dresses and cosmetics for himself, making him her confidante, and being the central figure in his life to the exclusion of father. Simply said, both parents show their son the 'benefits' of being homosexual; the father by being an ineffectual male object and making masculinity unpalatable, the mother also making masculinity distasteful by being a more-than-effective female. The son in his turn *rarely ever aggresses towards his mother*. To challenge her powers, to disown his sole source of love, however spurious, would be unheard of. This, as a matter of fact, is one of the homosexual's prime problems and conflicts.

It is *both* parents' rejection of him, but in particular Emma's, and then Edward's subsequent retaliation, that is of major significance. It seems to show, in no uncertain terms, how detached he was from both these people and thus from any sort of sexual identity. The likelihood is that he was truly impotent, truly asexual and unable to relate to any human on any human level, both because of his childhood (mis)treatment and in his need to protect himself from that very (re)occurrence devoid of feelings of attachment and affection towards anything or anyone.

His devotion to his Lord is not an exception to the above but only a further affirmation. Where else can someone obtain such a deep feeling of strength and protection without the more common 'hazards' and strains of marriage, friendship, etc? His fervid embrace of the Almighty gave him the strength that he so lacked; yet the 'over-intensity' of it likewise underscored his deep deficits.

And yet with all of this, the parental rejection he must have experienced, his retaliation against it, his over-emphasis on his heavenly inheritance, in the final count Edward was truly his parent's child. With his childhood-past as an almost integral part of his molecular structure he knew, in his bones, how to be both mother and father *without deviation*. On one level he really had no other woman above his mother; and is not an abstract Lord a fitting replacement for an abstract father? Is it also too far-fetched to compare his treatment of his 'subject-children' with that which he received at his parents' knees? Did he not, when it truly mattered, exile (abandon) his 'children' unto a foreign country; did he not treat his 'children' with weakness *and* parsimony in depriving them of their country and an English king? Does it not seem that, king though he was, he functioned with the same basic motives that most humans do, namely: to do right by his parents, to grow up to be like them, and to remain his parents' good little boy?

Such was the complicated man, ruler of a kingdom in chaos but himself enjoying a fleeting political triumph and a rare freedom of mind, whom Duke William came to see in 1051 to obtain a recommendation that he should be the next King of England. The circumstances were, of course, highly favourable to William's diplomacy and it would have been entirely out of keeping with his habitual astuteness if he had not used them. Edward was in a mood to listen to anything William wanted to say. He was master in his own house, not subject to Godwin's dictation but free to do and say what he pleased. Nobody knows what passed between Edward and William, for no records were kept and no scribes of the time wrote a word that has survived about any transaction between them. However, since there is evidence in plenty of Edward's partiality towards William and to Normandy, it may be reasonably supposed that William did secure some kind of promise regarding the throne of England. Two points are to be made about this. It is irrelevant to decide whether any such promise was made because (a) the crown was not Edward's to give away since, as we have noted, it was the Witan which had the right of choice; and (b) any recommendation by Edward did not remotely imply a hereditary right to the succession.

When he got home, William set about side-stepping these obstacles. Within two years he had married into the royal blood line of England. The wife he chose was Mathilda, a daughter of Count Baldwin of Flanders and a descendant of King Alfred the Great of England. The marriage by no means put William into a favourite's place in the succession, but it helped his cause. It is illustrative of the close bonds of kinship within the ruling families of England and northern Europe that Mathilda was a sister-in-law of Tostig, one of Godwin's sons. It is further illustrative of these links that William and Mathilda were of such near relationship (Mathilda's mother, Adele, was William's aunt) that their union trespassed the limits of consanguinity prescribed by the Church of Rome in 1049. Pope Leo condemned the marriage, but within six years William had attended to that impediment to his ambition. Pope Leo died and William thereupon approached the new Pope, Nicholas II, for a dispensation sanctioning the obviously successful union. Nicholas favoured the pious, temperate and powerful duke, to whom, as we shall see, he gave the blessing of the Church in 1066 regarding the climatic enterprise of William's life. In 1059 the bargain over the sanctioning of the marriage was agreeably closed with a promise that both William and Mathilda would found a church in Normandy as monuments to themselves and the benignity of Rome. The abbeys of St Etienne and La Trinité in Caen stand today as reminders of this promise. William's foundation of St Etienne became known as *L'Abbaye aux Hommes* and Mathilda's as *L'Abbaye aux Dames.* She was buried there and still rests in the choir. William was buried in his abbey and lay there until 1562, when enraged Huguenots dug up and scattered his bones during their revolt against the religious establishment of France.

Although the marriage was of course one in which diplomacy took precedence over emotion, it was always a conspicuously happy one until Mathilda died in 1083, four years before William. A strong contributing reason for the rare felicity was that William was unlike most members of the Norman feudal hierarchy in that he was no womaniser or high-flying wassailer. Professor Barlow suggests that William's sexual impulses might have been curbed by his bitter appreciation of how unrestrained sexuality on the part of his own father had branded him as illegitimate. William's son and successor, Rufus, was a notorious homosexual.

Implied confirmation that William had at least not inherited his father's appreciative eye for a pretty woman is offered by the fact that Mathilda was apparently close to being a physical freak, albeit a fruitful one. Her total progeny was four sons (two of whom became Kings of England and one a Duke of Normandy) and at least five daughters. But when her coffin in her church of Holy Trinity in Caen was opened and her bones examined in 1961 the startling discovery was made, according to Professor Michel de Bouard of the University of Caen, that she could not have been more than 50 inches tall – dwarflike even in an age when men and women were as a whole somewhat shorter than those living today in Europe and even shorter than the milk-fed giants of North America.*

Whatever the strength or weakness of William's sexual drives, they were subordinate to a far more powerful impulse which thrust him onwards to the acquisition of power and the capture of one of the pleasantest, and potentially one of the richest, islands in the world of his day.

Harold – Warrior Earl

Harold Godwinson was 44 in 1066, six years older than William and probably at the peak of his physical powers and military acumen. He was the more experienced field warrior of the two but,

* See Appendix A, p. 191.

as our narrative will disclose, the lesser strategist, in spite of his added maturity. He seems to have exhibited much more of the rough and tough Viking than William. He was only two generations removed from his Danish origins and he had grown up in an island which for all its closeness to Europe was very much a place apart – a kingdom whose people felt themselves (as do their successors of today) to be quite different from 'those foreigners' occupying the great land mass only 21 miles away at its nearest point. The temperamental stretch of water marking the separation had already been for many centuries far more effective than any land frontier in inhibiting fraternization; and strife, between continental and insular tribesmen and now in the eleventh century, had caused many of the islanders to be more conservative and less advanced in their thinking and habits of life than the Europeans.

Harold's father became so dominant in the island that in 1051 he could challenge his king for control of the kingdom, but he was a man of low and obscure social origins. Godwin's own father was Wolfnoth, a Danish warrior-pirate who came to England in one of the Viking raids which tormented the country during the disastrous reign of Ethelred the Unready, and he eventually settled in the southern shire of Sussex, almost certainly near Bosham. Godwin may have been low-born, but he had the fire of aggressive energy burning within him and was also a natural leader and a guileful politician. He was an early example of the self-made man, the type who will always rise, from no matter what base birth. As he did so, he shrewdly advanced his own status, first by choosing as his wife Gytha the sister of a Viking earl and a cousin of King Canute, and then by coaxing or coercing Edward the Confessor into marrying his daughter, Edith. He is believed to have done so not only to promote the interests of the House of Godwin directly but also to divert Edward from opening the door of England still wider to Norman intrusion by marrying one of its noble daughters.

Godwin did not live to see his son crowned king, but when he died in 1053 he knew that Harold would certainly succeed him as the virtual ruler of the kingdom in the name of King Edward, for there seemed to be nobody in England standing in his way to the throne when Edward died. That Harold eventually did so, albeit briefly and tragically, was as much a tribute to the extraordinary pertinacity of the father as to the quieter but equally effective exercise of authority by the son. The rise of the House of Godwin until its total obliteration in 1066 was the more remarkable because none of its members boasted one drop of English royal blood and it had no title whatever to the throne. Harold's condition as a commoner was of considerable importance to his fortunes in 1066. William could and did play upon this disadvantage in the preliminary propaganda skirmishes to the great clash of arms; and Englishmen with no particular feelings of loyalty to the House of Godwin, or bearing enmity or jealousy towards it, could salve their consciences by telling themselves that they need have no pangs of guilt in refusing to fight for a man without the usual valid right to the throne he occupied. There is evidence pointing to such backsliding.

Physically, Harold was a little shorter than William, but probably rather more solidly built. His record as a fighter in the field suggests that he also had more animal strength and stamina than William, whose feats as a warrior were constantly magnified beyond credibility by his scribes. But both men would today be regarded as of marvellous prowess and endurance – a little shorter and stockier than the men of today but far more muscular and trim. Both had grown up in an era when daily life was arduous even for the rich and privileged, and survival depended upon physical toughness. Normans and Englishmen of those days would have found the modern European or American an unbelievable namby-pamby with his central heating, soft bed, packaged food around the corner or within easy ride by the muscle-binding motor car; and the aeroplane, train and fuelled ship to take him effortlessly across the world. Familiar to them were the hard wooden bench, the back of a short-legged pony, smoking and reeking homes, smelly bodies, and no trained doctor or potent drug to succour them if they fell ill. They lived close to the earth, men with only primitive defences against the swift and mostly harsh caprices of nature. Harold's boyhood and youth had been more physically exacting than William's, for life in the island on the northern shore of the Channel was even more rugged than among the Normans, who had profited for generations from the readier exchange of ideas and devices with the peoples of the many European duchies and states bordering their territory. Moreover, the climate of England was then, as now, damper and more raw and consequently more demanding during most months of the year.

Harold had met and survived all the challenges since his birth

in 1022 and in so doing had developed a courage and resourcefulness outstanding in a period when these qualities were widespread.
Even the Bayeux Tapestry, dedicated as it was to proving him
an oath-breaker and a usurper, goes out of its way to emphasize
his gallantry – principally, we must deduce, to elevate William's
ultimate triumph, but also because Harold *was* militarily heroic.
Several panels of the Tapestry are used to tell of his bravery in
rescuing two soldiers from quicksands while riding with William
during a minor campaign in Brittany. The episode is depicted as
having occurred while Harold was making that mysterious visit to
William's court. We may justifiably dispute much of the message
which the Tapestry is intended to convey, but there seems no good
reason to disbelieve that some such incident as the rescue of the
soldiers did occur at some time; it would be an odd event for
somebody to invent.

It is also in keeping with accounts of other instances of Harold's
physical courage. Thus, the scribe in the Anglo-Saxon Chronicle
records that in one military engagement as a young man Harold
'fought most resolutely' (a phrase which perhaps indicates that the
English habit of under-statement was already established 900
years ago), and all versions of the Chronicle stress the thoroughness
and spirit with which he carried through one of his most memorable missions on behalf of Edward the Confessor – the subjugation
of Griffith, a rebellious Welsh sub-king, two years before the
Battle of Hastings. Harold's onslaught against Griffith was so
determined that the Welsh warriors whom it sent reeling back into
their mountain encampments turned there upon Griffith, their
leader. They cut off his head and sent it as a grisly but incon-
trovertible token of surrender to Harold's command post. In turn,
he took it back with him to Winchester to prove to Edward the
completion of his mission. Harold did not escape Welsh family
vengeance for his defeat and disposal of Griffith. A year later
the dead sub-king's son, Caradoc, swooped down upon a hunting
lodge which Harold, rather riskily, was having built on Welsh soil
at Portskewet, close to the point where today the Severn Tunnel
emerges at its western end. Caradoc's men ravaged the lodge, killing
almost all the men who were working on it and taking away as
much of the material lying there as they possibly could.

Harold's journey to manhood was much less hazardous than
William's, for he was no noble prince sitting upon, or as yet even

the heir to, a throne upon which others had designs. He grew up as the second of a brood of five boys and one girl under the more than adequate protection of a father who was thrusting ambitiously in many directions. Godwin continued to acquire land in England until his domain of Wessex stretched from Kent to Cornwall, forcing his will upon King Edward, and dominating the rival but cowed Earls Siward of Northumbria and Leofric of Mercia. Godwin's devotion to the furtherance of personal and family interests undoubtedly affected the character of his sons. It completely spoilt two of them – Sweyn, the eldest, and Tostig, the third son – and it appears to have taught Harold the valuable but dangerous truth that boldness usually yields the biggest rewards. Godwin certainly proved that might was right, in the disorganized island of England, divided under a weak king between a few quarrelling nobles. Godwin's methods of protecting himself and his power and of imposing his will upon his rivals were cruel, often diabolically savage by our standards, and much evidence survives to show that Harold copied his father, somewhat less extremely, while he was serving first as Godwin's right-hand man and afterwards as Earl of Wessex and the King's Chancellor. Harold took over from his father when the old man died hard, as he had lived, and in circumstances like those which marked the end of a similar self-made man and tyrant of the twentieth century, Joseph Stalin. He was cut down by a stroke while eating with his two sons, Harold and Tostig and the King, at Winchester on Easter Monday, 1053, one year after the banishment of the whole family had ended. He lingered until the following Thursday without recovering speech or movement. Harold succeeded him without challenge.

One cannot now detect when he first began to cherish thoughts and plans of succeeding the ageing Edward, but it seems quite likely that he was already doing so in collusion with Godwin long before his father died. A significant event in 1057 shows that he was certainly thinking along those lines in that year and it also raises the probability that he would not hesitate at murder to clear his path to the succession. In 1057 Edward Atheling, who, as a son of Edmund Ironsides (King of England for seven months in 1016) and a nephew of King Edward, was the next in line of succession to the throne, suddenly came back to the country from Hungary. He had been living there for 20 years after having been sent away by King Canute for some offence of which there is no historical record. One Saxon chronicler says obliquely and mysteriously that Canute sent him to Hungary 'in order to betray him', but the Atheling not only avoided whatever trap had been laid for him but prospered and married a princess of the royal Hungarian blood. His luck deserted him, however, when he arrived back in England. He died suspiciously suddenly while still in his mid-forties, not even surviving long enough to see his royal uncle. His fate was very like that of an earlier heir to the throne (Alfred, King Edward's brother) who, as we have seen, was almost certainly murdered by Godwin. Is it stretching calumny too far to suggest that Harold had something to do with the removal of the inconvenient Atheling in 1057? The Saxon chronicler surely had suspicions of some kind for he wrote that year with even more than usual wariness: 'We do not know for what reason it was brought about that he was not allowed to visit his kinsman King Edward. Alas, that was a miserable fate and grievous to all this people that he so speedily ended his life after he came to England, to the misfortune of this poor realm.' We must make of that entry what we can, for no satisfactory answers can be offered to the questions it raises. But of one fact there would appear to be no doubt at all – the scribe knew a great deal more than he wrote. Suspicion swings towards Harold in the affair for two reasons which, when considered together, show that he had much more to gain than anybody else from the removal of the Atheling. These were (a) that with the death of the Atheling there remained no direct hereditary heir to Edward the Confessor, and (b) that as the most powerful commoner in the land Harold stood in the best position to benefit from this circumstance when Edward died.

It would be foolish to maintain that Harold was much too noble to stoop to murder. He undoubtedly had the same scant regard for other peoples' lives as did most political and warrior leaders of his period. Even the inhabitants of his family's earldom were not spared when Harold was on his warpath. Thus, when he and his father contrived to end the winter of their banishment, to which Edward had sentenced them in 1051, Harold was merciless in crushing domestic opposition to his return. The Chronicle describes his father's arrival on the Isle of Wight from Bruges, in Belgium, and goes on: 'Meanwhile Harold was sailing from Ireland with nine ships and landed at Porlock, in Somerset, where many people were gathered to oppose him; but he did not hesitate to provide himself with food. He went inland and slew a great part of the inhabitants, including more than thirty good thanes besides other men, and seized whatever he pleased in cattle, captives and property.' This does not sound like the work of a man with scruples or with much compassion when pursuing a set military purpose; nor does it sound like that of a man who, as the Normans would have the world believe, tamely agreed to support the claim of a foreign duke to a throne which he clearly believed was to be his, and to which he acceded with what many Englishmen regarded in 1066 as unseemly haste after Edward the Confessor had died and was not yet buried.

Nevertheless, Harold served Edward loyally and efficiently during the last ten years of the reign. Recorded episodes other than the putting down of Griffith reflect his determination to preserve peace in the country. One episode especially seems to demonstrate that he was prepared to put the national well-being above the interests of the Godwin clan, although here again there is the hidden possibility that at the same time he was furthering his own purposes in the bargain. This was a drama in 1065 which led to the ousting of his brother, Tostig, as Earl of Northumbria. Faced with the choice of supporting his brother in a rampage of rampacity, cruelty and tyranny within his earldom, or serving king and people by subjecting Tostig to justice, Harold chose the latter. Perhaps the decision was not all that hard to make, for Tostig seems undoubtedly to have been cursed with more than a fair share of human baseness. He was spoilt, hot-tempered, cruel and vindictive, and Harold may well have felt that the removal of Tostig would strengthen his own position as well as national tranquillity.

Tostig was Earl of Northumbria for only one year but during that brief period of tenure he managed to make himself so detested that his people almost went to war to get rid of him. He had reverted to his Viking origins with a vengeance, gathering around him in Northumbria a band of ungodly Danes to support him in imposing a term of cruelty and plunder upon the people whom he was supposed to protect and lead. In the late summer of 1065 citizens in the towns and villages of the north united in organizing a rebellion against him because, as the annal states, he had 'robbed God first and then despoiled of life and land all those over whom he could tyrannize.' The rebels overran Tostig's military camp at York and after killing all his retainers whom they could find, 'whether English or Danish', seized everything available belonging to him there. They were taking advantage of one of Tostig's frequent visits to Edward's court in the south of England; he is reputed to have been out hunting with Edward in Hampshire when the revolt bloomed.

The rebels now invited Morcar, a brother of the neighbouring earl Edwin of Mercia, to take over Northumbria from Tostig. Once again England was faced with civil war as the Yorkshiremen, led by Morcar, marched south to join their forces with Edwin's and put the choice to King Edward : Give us Morcar in place of Tostig or meet us to fight it out. Men from Nottingham, Derby and Lincoln joined the rebellion and even bands of marauding Welshmen, ever willing to take advantage of English troubles, added themselves. Edward called on Harold for help and sent him to parley with the rebels at Oxford. Harold listened to their case against Tostig and evidently decided that even he should not, and probably could not, save his brother. He went back to Winchester to recommend to the king that Tostig should be outlawed and Morcar installed in his place. While he was doing so, the rebels demonstrated to Edward that he would be wise to accept the advice by capturing the town of Northampton, 40 miles from Oxford, and sacking it. Edward had no real choice in the matter for the rebels were obviously strong enough to overthrow him if he defied them. He sent Harold back for a second meeting with them amid the ruins of Northampton to say that he agreed to the change. On 27 October the rebels set out again for home, taking with them many captives and head of cattle. Harold had neither the forces nor presumably the wish to challenge them on this pillage. They had won, and the human and animal spoils were theirs.

Tostig fled the country with his wife and family and those of his retainers who had survived. He led them across the Channel to Calais and thereafter they settled at St Omer, some 20 miles inland, as the winter guests of the ever-receptive Count Baldwin of Flanders, Tostig's brother-in-law. Tostig promptly set about preparing to show Harold that if he thought he had improved his own position close to the throne by getting rid of his brother he was in grievous error. Like everybody else, Tostig knew that William of Normandy was preparing to claim the throne of England when Edward died without a direct heir, and he also knew that Edward was failing fast. A scene was being set in which Tostig could take his vengeance upon Harold. He did not have long to wait.

Edward died on 5 January 1066, before the winter was half over. Harold virtually seized the throne. On the very day that Edward was being buried at his new church and abbey at Westminster, Harold had himself proclaimed by a makeshift and debilitated Witan composed only of his friends and allies. One who did have a valid claim to the throne was summarily brushed aside. He was Edgar Atheling, son of the Edward Atheling who had died with such mysterious suddenness nine years earlier. Edgar was still a boy and there was nobody in authority who dared, or probably wished, to support him when Harold and his followers simply ignored him. It was no time to install a boy as King of England.

Although Harold's haste in taking control of the country does seem superficially to be suspicious, there were in fact some strong diplomatic reasons to explain it. Primarily, there was the hard fact that a man on a throne is immeasurably stronger and more difficult to challenge than one who waits to make a claim. Then there was Duke William who had already proclaimed for all to hear that he considered himself Edward's successor and would surely come to claim his inheritance. Harold's domestic situation also contained factors to spur him on. He could count upon a following only in the south, the south-west, and the south-east. He was himself already lord of the south and south-west and his control of the country south of a diagonal stretching roughly from Gloucester to the Wash was buttressed by the authority of two of his brothers. They were Leofwin, holding great areas of Kent, Surrey and other country close to London, and Gyrth, holding East Anglia.

The rest of the island was either lukewarm or hostile to him. Edwin and Morcar in the midlands of Mercia and the wilds of Northumbria owed him something for the removal of Tostig and the elevation to his earldom of Morcar, but they belonged to a noble house (founded by their grandfather Leofric of Mercia) which had long been at enmity with Godwin and whose power had actually been enhanced by Morcar's accession. Harold could not expect the brothers now to accept him with enthusiasm as their non-royal king and overlord. So he simply gave them no time to come south and make trouble for him at the Witan. Nor did he wish to give the feverishly nationalistic and hostile Welsh an opportunity to march again against him. Finally, he could expect nothing from the

Scots north of the Tweed. They had secured their independence from England half a century earlier, and a punitive campaign against them in 1054, in answer to many border raids against Northumbria, had failed to shake that independence although it had deposed the usurper Macbeth and installed the exiled Malcolm as King of the Cumbrians.

It is not surprising then that Harold was in such a hurry to get himself crowned. The haste was noted, of course, in Normandy and it provided more useful propaganda for William against Harold. In this connection, it is to be noted that the Bayeux Tapestry deliberately misrepresented the coronation. It shows, and declares, that Stigand, Archbishop of Canterbury, crowned Harold whereas all the reliable contemporary English chroniclers state unequivocally that the ceremony was performed by Aldred, Archbishop of York. The naming of Stigand, a notorious cleric, was intended to give the impression, it would seem, that Harold chose one of his unworthy cronies to crown him – an archbishop who was formally deposed by five successive popes and was not trusted by most of his fellow prelates. The designers of the Tapestry cannot reasonably be excused as having made a genuine mistake.

One other weakness marred Harold's position as king. He had no queen, with useful family connections, to sit beside him on the throne. He did not waste much time, however, in filling this gap, for early in 1066 (the exact date has never been determined) he sought to mend a lot of fences by marrying Aldyth, a sister of Edwin and Morcar, and the widow of the Griffith whom he had destroyed only three years ago.

The marriage, like King Edward's, was loveless and barren, but for different reasons. It could scarcely have been otherwise, for long before Harold became king he had taken to himself a permanent mistress who had borne him several sons and two daughters. She is an obscure figure in history. The references to her in the various chronicles and formal documents of the period are vague and brief. They confirm her existence as a woman of position and property but, alas, they do not tell us anything of her personality or her influence upon Harold and the events of his period. She is known to us, vaguely and romantically, as Edith of the Swan Neck.

This name, written in the vernacular as 'Edgyva Swanneshals', is the only one by which she is ever mentioned directly. But there is some inferential evidence to suggest that she was a native of

Norfolk. In the Chronicle of John of Oxenides, written after 1292, her name appears in a list of benefactors to the Abbey of St Benet of Holm, to which she apparently gave the village of Thurgarton, Norfolk. The gift was confirmed by King Edward in 1046 and is recorded in the Domesday Survey. Elsewhere in Domesday, a mistress of Harold (*quaedam concubina Haraldi*) is mentioned as holding three houses in Canterbury, in Harold's earldom, and in view of the long association between the two it is believed that this woman is almost certainly Edith Swan Neck – even though the spiteful and voluble William of Poitiers accuses Harold of being guilty of 'abominable riotous living' (*luxuria foedus*).

Harold's Spirited Daughter

Some valid if incidental deductions are to be made from this disparate evidence. Since Edith Swan Neck was already a property owner of importance in Norfolk in 1046, she was probably in her forties by the time of Harold's accession and the Battle of Hastings. She was not, however, far beyond the child-bearing age, for she had one illegitimate daughter by Harold who was only three or four years old when her father lost his throne and his life at Hastings. She was named Gunhilda and was to provide what must have been a major scandal in England in the last decade of the century. Like other spirited women of the period – such as Arletta of Falaise and her daughter, and Emma, the mother of Edward the Confessor – she broke through the confines imposed by men to keep the female sex in what they considered to be its proper place.

After the battle of Hastings she was taken by her mother to join other high-born Anglo-Saxon women and children at a monastery at Wilton, in Wiltshire, which was for a long time to provide sanctuary as the Normans overran the country and then started governing and reorganizing it. There Gunhilda grew up in safety and seclusion. As an adolescent she took the veil but did not make the formal profession which would have dedicated her to lifetime service of Christ. Something, perhaps an instinctive urge for freedom, prompted her not to take the final, irrevocable step. Gunhilda must have been a lovely woman, or at least one with that indefinable aura of femininity which draws men to her type. Nothing is known about any romantic associations she might have had while she was still a young woman, but she certainly made some startling conquests thereafter. In 1093, 27 years after the battle and when she would be about 30 years old, she dramatically conquered Count Alan Rufus, the lord of Richmond (Yorkshire) and the most powerful Norman aristocrat in northern England. Alan Rufus went to the nunnery at Wilton to claim as his wife Mathilda, a daughter of Malcolm King of Scots. In the rather heartless fashion of the times Malcolm had promised her, a girl of 13, to Alan Rufus, a man in his middle fifties. The ill-balanced union was not to be, for Alan Rufus saw Gunhilda in the nunnery, and was evidently captivated by her. He rejected Mathilda and claimed Gunhilda. In all probability the child Mathilda knew little or nothing of the jilting; it certainly did her no harm in the marriage market, for she later married King Henry I (1100–1135) and flourished as a Queen of England and Duchess of Normandy. But the romance between Alan Rufus and Gunhilda was brief and unfulfilled. They went off to the north of England presumably hoping to share a life of power and plenty. Death disposed otherwise. Alan Rufus died on 4 August 1093, before they were even married. Gunhilda did not retire decorously to the nunnery at Wilton. She became instead the consort, though probably not the wife, of Alan Rufus's brother who had succeeded to the family titles and lands and apparently to his brother's other possessions as well.

Gunhilda's wanton behaviour is reckoned to have caused a national scandal. Above all it scandalized the head of the English church, Anselm, who that same year had become Archbishop of Canterbury and was showing himself to be one of the most devoted and keen-minded clerics of the early Middle Ages. But Anselm was also a man. He had met Gunhilda some years earlier in the nunnery, probably in 1086, and had never forgotten her. He was shocked when she went off so readily with Alan Rufus. He wrote her a letter which speaks much for the complexes and suppressions in the mind of an enforced celibate, a godly man who was later to become a saint of the Roman church. The letter survives as one of the few relics from the establishment at Wilton. It reads :

Receive, dearest and most longed-for daughter, receive these words to the honour of God and to your own great benefit as an admonition of your true lover. [One must believe that he meant not himself but Jesus Christ.] You once spoke to me and said you wished to be ever with me so that you could enjoy an un-interrupted talk. You said you found it sweet; and you afterwards wrote me a letter full of sweetness in which I could see that you would not renounce the holy profession of which you then wore the habit. I hoped you would fulfil what you promised in God's name.

This letter, so full of meaning and so pent in its terms, clearly did nothing to curb Gunhilda's lust for the full life outside the nunnery. She went her way and provoked Anselm to write her again in savage terms, after Alan Rufus had died but just before she made the alliance with his brother. The letter read (according to J. Southern, who translated it in 1936):

You loved Count Rufus and he you. Where is he now? What has become of the lover you once loved? Go now and lie with him in the bed where he now lies; gather his worms into your bosom; embrace his corpse; kiss his bare teeth from which the flesh has fallen. He does not now care for your love in which he delighted while he lived; and the flesh which you desired now rots.

Anselm was undoubtedly writing to Gunhilda primarily as her Archbishop to reproach her because she had abandoned love of Christ for the impure and ephemeral love of man. But do not the harsh terms of the letter, considered in relation to his earlier missive, show that he might also have been writing as a man? Might there not have been purely personal bitterness and perhaps some jealousy exercising him as he painted in such extreme phrases the frustration of Gunhilda's carnal hopes?

Nothing is known about Gunhilda's life after she joined the brother of Alan Rufus until as an old woman she did eventually go back into obscurity at Wilton. There is a final reference to her in surviving records. William of Malmesbury, a prolific and imaginative writer who flourished in the first half of the twelfth century, tells an appropriate story about this spectacular daughter of King Harold. In a book in which he describes miracles supposedly achieved by Wulfstan, who was Bishop of Worcester between 1062 and 1095 and was later made a saint, he says that Wulfstan visited Wilton and cured Gunhilda of a tumour of the eye as she languished there towards the end of her days.

Gunhilda had a sister, Gytha, whose career was much less lively. She is believed to have been sent to safety in Denmark soon after the Conquest and, according to the Scandanavian saga writers, she eventually became the wife of Vladimir, a Prince of Novgorod. Although Gytha's earthly career was so much less conspicuous than her sister's, her place in history is far more significant. Through her, Queen Elizabeth II is descended from Harold. The authority for this fascinating connection is Patrick Montague-Smith, the genealogist. Writing as assistant editor of *Debrett*, he explained to readers of the *Daily Telegraph* on 11 November 1961, that one son of Gytha and Prince Vladimir (named Mistislav Harold) was a forebear of Philippa of Hainault, who became the queen of Edward III of England (1327–1377). Thus, the blood-link between Queen Elizabeth and King Harold is thin, but it apparently exists, thanks to Gytha.

3

The Challengers Prepare

News of Edward's death and Harold's prompt coup in seizing the vacant throne was known within a week in the three centres of eleventh century civilization to which it was of prime importance – northern Europe, Rome and Scandinavia. The full story reached Tostig in St Omer in about three days and it probably came to Duke William in Normandy only a short time later. It would reach Rome, of which England was a spiritual ward and a wayward one into the bargain, at about the same moment as it was taken by ship to Norway, where King Harald Hardrada, one of the legendary warrior figures of the era, was weighing *his* chances of annexing a land which had long been linked forcibly and otherwise with Scandinavia. The exit of King Edward the Confessor without an indisputable heir had left England a likely prey to men of hungry character – William, Tostig and Harald Hardrada. William and Harald Hardrada each wanted it for himself; Tostig wanted vengeance upon his brother.

Harold Godwinson needed desperately to strengthen his shaky hold upon his kingdom with all speed, in order to meet the onslaughts which he knew would surely be made upon him as soon as they could be prepared. He had little solid foundation upon which to build his claim to the loyalty of Englishmen beyond the prestige of the House of Godwin and his physical possession of power in the critical areas of the south of England. He had no valid right to the throne and he had no English royal blood in his veins – only the thinnest trickle of foreign royal blood because on his mother's side going back three generations he was a descendant of Harold Blotand, who had been King of Denmark from 935 until 985.

His realm in 1066 was nothing like the cohesive unit it was to become many decades later. It was not even as unified as Alfred the Great had left it in 899. Among his successors, Ethelred the Unready (who reigned for an unusually long period between 979 and 1016) had probably done most to cause Alfred's work and his inspiration to wither. Ethelred had succeeded his brother, Edward, who was murdered by unknown assailants at Corfe, in Dorset. Throughout his kingship he confirmed the superstitious fears which arose in the year of his coronation at Kingston-on-Thames when 'a cloud red as blood was seen, frequently with the appearance of fire, and it usually appeared about midnight.' Worse still, people got to know that at Ethelred's christening he had defiled the font. This mishap caused Dunstan, Archbishop of Canterbury, to forecast with dark accuracy that such an infant would achieve little good during his lifetime. Ethelred and his advisers showed chronic feebleness in running the country and, particularly, in meeting the Vikings who exploited weakness by making a series of invasions. The contemporary scribes fill the Anglo-Saxon Chronicle with accounts of the invaders' depredations against a more or less undefended land, and one of them says bitterly in his account of the year 1010: 'And when the enemy was in the east, then our levies were mustered in the west; and when they were in the south, then our levies were in the north.' Three years later Wulfstan, Archbishop of York, recounted the evils of the times in a sermon in which he deplored the destruction of citizens' rights and even the sale of adults and children into slavery. Canute had made amends for Ethelred, but Harold's immediate predecessor, Edward the Confessor, had restored division and unrest by packing his court, church and state with foreign Norman favourites.

Anglo-Saxon England had been like a man who takes a few steps forward and then takes a big one backwards. This had been so for some ten centuries, since the time when a quarter of a million Celts had lived in little more than one-fifth of the country – and, it has been coldly recorded, ceremonially ate some of their womenfolk at Salmonby, in Gloucestershire. Succeeding generations of invading and victorious tribes had made many strides from the depths of such savagery, but there had been disquieting relapses. Some of them had happened not so very long before Harold became King and should be remembered whenever we are tempted to over-estimate the extent of civilization and sophistication in the England of his day. The limitations had been signalled by events such as the pelting to death with bones and the skulls of cattle of a Bishop of London by rampaging Vikings in 1012, half a century before Harold became King. More recently the savage beheading of Griffith by his own men had occurred when they were beaten by Harold in the mountains in 1063.

Even after the Conquest violence and the prosecution of family feuds continued. They included some which had lasted for generations in Anglo-Saxon days. For example, one feud which had begun in Northumbria in 1016 between the houses of two nobles, Uchtred and Thorbrand, was bloodily revived some years after William became king. A descendant of Uchtred avenged the original murder of his grandfather, which had started the feud, by leading a raid upon the sons of the murderer while they were feasting at Settrington, killing everybody except two diners who managed to flee into the woods.

Harold now turned his attention in these early days of 1066 firstly to the two brother earls, Edwin and Morcar, who between them controlled those parts of England which he did not. He needed at the very least their passive neutrality in the coming struggles with William, Tostig and Harald Hardrada; at best he might get pledges of help from them in the form of soldiers and supplies. He rode north in the early spring of 1066 primarily to win over to his side, with the help of his friend, Bishop Wulfston, some settlements which had shown a threat of rebellion. While in Mercia and Northumbria he talked with Edwin and Morcar. The nature and outcome of these talks is unknown, but it is considered highly probable by historians that during this visit he married Aldyth, their sister, as part of his strategy to gain their goodwill. Judging by the spiritless and inglorious part played by the brothers in the coming avalanche of events during the rest of the year, the move was a total failure. Aldyth became Harold's queen but she did not become his wife; that role had been occupied for many years by Edith Swan Neck, and she was unlikely to be ousted now by an ageing widow of some 40 years who had been picked up so calculatingly by Harold as a pawn in his domestic diplomacy.

Like Harold, William lost no time in confirming that he was in deadly earnest about claiming England for himself. As soon as he heard what had happened at the turn of the year he sent a series of angry and threatening messages to Harold. They claimed that Harold had usurped a throne to which William was the true heir and in so doing had betrayed a solemn oath sworn on holy relics at William's court. No matter whether these charges were true or false they formed a base upon which William could – and did – build a case for justification of his invasion. These blistering messages were probably verbal ones carried across the Channel by Norman couriers, for no written record of William's words has survived anywhere, and the use of human messengers (bodes, as they were called) was usual in those times. Like most military leaders of medieval days, Harold and William were illiterate and accordingly relied far more frequently upon the spoken than the written word for their communications. Neither is there any written evidence of what Harold said or wrote in rebuttal of William's accusations. But a curious extension of the story of Harold's oath to William was produced some 40 years later by Eadmer, a monk serving as an assistant to Archbishop Anselm. Eadmer had heard a tale that as part of a bargain reached between William and Harold in Normandy William gave one of his young daughters in betrothal to Harold. She has since been identified as Agatha, one of five or six daughters born to William and Mathilda. She eventually died unmarried. She must have been at least pre-adolescent in 1066, but even infants were sometimes formally betrothed in the eleventh century. (Agatha's own maternal grandmother had been betrothed as a child to Duke Richard the Third of Normandy and had to be kept for several years at a relative's court in Flanders until the marriage could respectably take place and be consummated.) Eadmer plainly doubted the story of Agatha's betrothal to Harold and goes out of his way to clear Harold's memory in connection with it. He repeats a widely-held belief that the girl had anyhow died before Harold came to the throne and he argues that even had she lived Harold, as a king, could not be held to any promise of marriage to her. Writing some 600 years later, John Milton reproduces this argument, saying : 'Harold could not take her now as an outlandish (i.e. foreign) woman without the consent of the realm.'

Harold had been king only three months when he had to face the first probing challenge from across the Channel. It was a sortie from Flanders by his brother Tostig and was particularly ominous since it indicated that Tostig was operating in collusion with Duke William. In all probability the pair had been in touch with each other during the winter and, although there is naturally no record of any firm arrangement between them, it would seem certain that, as soon as they heard that Edward had died and Harold had succeeded him, they formed an alliance by which Tostig would draw Harold's fire, as it were, on the promise of rewards to come when William had conquered England.

Tostig put out from Flanders early in April with a fleet carrying a force of his own Housecarls (household troops) and made an unopposed landing on the Isle of Wight, probably at Winstone, just outside the modern town of Shanklin. It is a sign of the unsettled state of England as well as an indication of Harold's uncertain hold upon the people of his kingdom that the Wight islanders actually welcomed his fraternal challenger. They gave him money and provisions and doubtless other forms of sustenance before he sailed off on an expedition of plunder, despoliation and harassment on a long stretch of the English southern coast, much of it opposite Normandy, between Portsmouth and the south-easterly approaches to London. Harold wisely interpreted Tostig's raids as preliminary probings to the well-advertised coming invasion by William. By the time Tostig had mauled coastal settlements of Sussex and Kent as far east as Sandwich, Harold had mobilized what the Anglo-Saxon Chronicle described as 'greater naval and land levies than any king in the country had ever gathered before, because he was credibly informed that William the Bastard* was about to invade this land to conquer it.'

Tostig played the traditional role of the guerilla fighter, darting briefly into action as opportunity offered and always avoiding a confrontation with a stronger enemy. He made off before Harold's army and navy could descend upon him. With his own forces augmented by some volunteers and unwilling conscripts rounded up in ports he had attacked, he left Sandwich and sailed northwards in 60 ships, up the North Sea via the coast of East Anglia and the Wash. He paused from time to time to make hit-and-run raids upon the thinly-peopled areas of north Lincolnshire now supporting the great cities of Lincoln and Grimsby and the boroughs of Cleethorpes, Louth and Scunthorpe. Then he sailed into the estuary of the river Humber to continue his harryings in territories belonging to Edwin of Mercia and Morcar of Northumbria, where he had so recently misgoverned as earl.

Harold was too experienced a general to swallow the bait so pointedly dangled by Tostig. He did not swing his forces northwards

---

* Another edition of the Chronicle describes William as 'kinsman of King Edward'. This is the version written at Abingdon and here, as elsewhere, it shows its anti-Godwin bias.

to chase after Tostig but held them in the south to muster them to the best advantage against the greater looming menace of William's invasion. He calculated that even if Edwin and Morcar would not support him as their King, and their wayward brother-in-law, they would at least defend their own possessions against the piratical and vengeful Tostig.

Harold ignored the earlier evidence of the coolness towards him in the Isle of Wight. He could do so safely. The total population probably numbered less than 1,000 and was divided into tiny settlements more or less isolated from each other, and so the islanders could by no means be reckoned as a threat to him. Accordingly, he took no account of them in using the south-eastern coast of the island, which jutted out far into the Channel, as the best possible base for his ships while they awaited William. He kept his fleet poised there to intercept any invading ships before they reached the English coast. He would have a good chance of crippling or sinking some of them, perhaps a decisive proportion, if he could get his navy into the close grapple with them. But he must also count upon the possibility that the wily William might be able to elude him and descend unweakened upon the coast. As a precaution he called up the fyrd, or militia, in the southern shires of his former earldom of Wessex and in the smaller earldoms of his younger brothers. He stationed these troops strategically at intervals on those parts of the coast where Tostig had cast a meaningful shadow in the early spring. But these soldiers were mostly untrained peasants and small farmers and Harold could not expect them to be able to withstand on their own an assault by William's knights and trained troops. Accordingly he stiffened their ranks with some of his own formidable Housecarls, to maintain their morale and to give them useful training while they awaited the enemy.

It was now close to high summer. Harold obviously believed that he could expect William to move at any moment. He had done all he could as a seasoned and skilful military commander to prepare for the coming blow. All things considered it would suit him well if William came soon.

Meanwhile, William had also been getting ready with his customary prudence and thoroughness. Tostig had served him well. To the hard-minded William, he was the more valuable because he was so obviously expendable, an ally whom William could coldly cast aside, if he survived, after his usefulness was over.

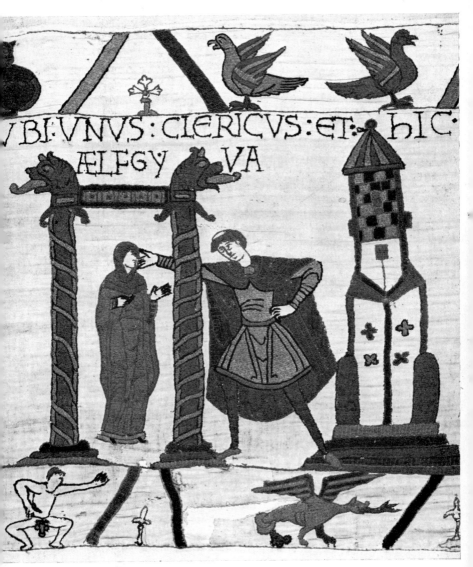

Part of the Bayeux Tapestry showing the mysterious Aelfgyva and the clergyman. In the lower border a naked figure apes the posture of the clothed man above.
Photo Phaidon Press.

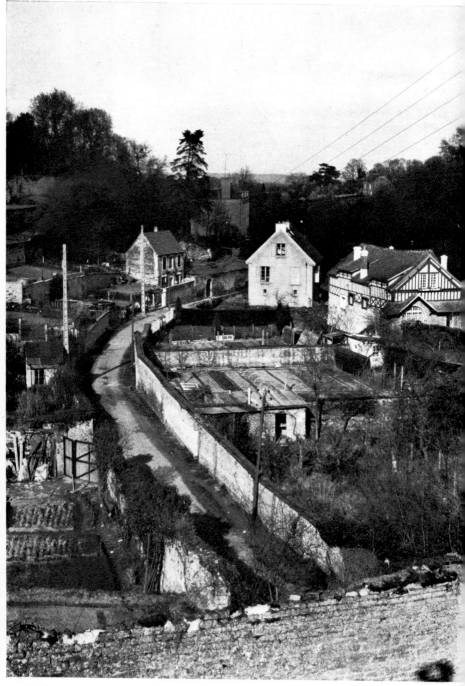

2 Falaise, Normandy, where Duke Robert the Devil met Arletta, the mother of William the Conqueror, has not changed greatly since the eleventh century.

Since William was nowhere near ready to make his own invasion in the spring, Tostig was of course doing him a most useful service in raiding England without establishing himself as a rival conquerer. He was not only challenging Harold's defences but causing them to be put into the field very early in the year; and this was to prove costly indeed to Harold before the year was out. With his small force of some 60 ships and several hundred men Tostig had not the remotest chance of establishing himself in England, even if such an ambition were flowering in his mind. Even with the unexpected addition of an ally who now joined him, Tostig did not emerge as either a rival to William or a danger to Harold. An independent pirate called Copsi, a thegn of Northumbria who had been one of Tostig's associates and deputies when Tostig was earl and who had probably been exiled at the same time as his lord, now entered the picture. He had fled northwards from Northumbria and had spent the winter in the Orkneys. Early in 1066 he started harrying coastal regions of England with a band of fellow pirates whom he had gathered about him during his winter of exile. Somewhere and somehow, probably by chance, he and Tostig met at sea and the pair promptly joined forces. Copsi's 15 ships and some 1,200 warriors and seamen helped to offset the losses which Tostig had incurred during his sorties against the English coasts, besides adding to the damage which the raiders could do.

William's Aims

The recital in the official records of Normandy for 1066 of what William did during the first six months of the year testify to his skill and the successes which it brought as he prepared his expedition. He had three principal aims at this stage of the enterprise:

1. To gather domestic and European support for the invasion and, if possible, to mask the sheer aggression behind the façade of a crusade approved by the Church of Rome.

2. To mass his knights, soldiers and ships at some suitable starting point for the Channel crossing, and provide them with all the equipment necessary to carry them through the first days of a difficult and dangerous land campaign in England.

C

3. To secure the tranquillity of Normandy while he was away on a mission from which he might never return and to establish an orderly succession to his throne in case he did not do so.

William set about his first task by holding a sequence of assemblies and conferences throughout his Duchy and by despatching emissaries to the royal courts of France and Flanders, and to Rome. One of his most successful ambassadors was Gilbert, Archdeacon of Lisieux, who went to Rome and obtained not only a formal legal judgement in favour of William's claim to the English throne but a public declaration by Pope Alexander III of the blessing of the Church upon the 'crusade'. It was a one-sided performance. There is no evidence that Harold or one of his representatives was invited to defend him against the accusations and arguments of the Archdeacon, and the regrettable conclusion must be drawn that the dealings between William and the papacy were strictly business-like and mutually self-serving. In return for a guarantee by William that he would bring an errant England firmly within the Catholic fold, Alexander agreed to give William all the moral support he needed to influence the fighting men of Normandy and northern Europe to join him in his expedition against Harold and England. The Pope had a lot to gain and nothing to lose by the arrangement. And William's chances of success were substantially improved by the papal approval in an era when the Church had such authority over men's lives and minds.

William's spokesman in Rome could easily make an exaggerated case against the inferior condition of the Church in England and the need for reform, for there were some notorious abuses and omissions in its performance. And since Christianity under the banner of Rome was the most powerful political and unifying force in Europe, William's shrewdly-emphasized contention that he would rescue England was heard with respect not only in Rome but in most of the continental states to which it was addressed. But to blame Harold for the shortcomings of the English Church was unjustified. He had been king for only a matter of weeks and in that short period he had been much too occupied in confirming his authority over a portion of a severely divided country threatened with invasion to be able to give any attention to Church reform.

One ecclesiastical blemish was that Stigand, a friend of the Godwin family but a churchman of highly dubious religious morality, was still Archbishop of Canterbury and Bishop of Winchester at one and the same time. Another imperfection was that the sale of Church appointments (simony) was being practised and that some of the clergy were openly immoral. Yet Harold had already given one sign that if he had reigned longer he might have made some reforms : he had had himself crowned in January by Aldred, Archbishop of York and a churchman of unsullied repute, instead of by Stigand, the premier archbishop. William's propagandists chose, as we have noted, not to acknowledge this quite significant action.

The fact that the church in England was not so corrupt as the Normans claimed is demonstrated by the innumerable and often irrelevant references made to the Church's authority and activity in the Anglo-Saxon Chronicle up to 1066. These references include quite a number of visits to Rome paid by Church leaders and their representatives and by secular pilgrims. But the distorted picture painted by Norman writers was unfortunately, and unworthily, reproduced wholesale several centuries later by John Milton in an effort to prove that England was conquered by William because of the sins of the English. Milton seems to have gone much too far in writing : 'Not many years before the Normans came the Clergy could scarcely read and understand their Latin service. He was a Miracle to others who knew his Grammar. The Monks went about in fine stuffs and made no difference what they ate; which though in itself no fault, yet to their Consciences was irreligious.'

The common people certainly supported their Church staunchly and practically. Over 400 churches still in use today in England have remnants of Anglo-Saxon construction in their fabrics and thereby give witness to the sturdiness of the work done. Design and architecture may have been crude but the labour was well-qualified. One of the most conspicuous monuments to public devotion in the eleventh century is the tower of All Saints Church at Earls Barton (Buartone in the Domesday survey) in Northamptonshire. It is a solid-looking tower made of stone and rubble with a protective outer covering of plaster and it has survived the batterings of ten centuries of English weather without losing its integrity. Experts have put its date of construction at 1070 and they assume that it served the dual purpose of a place of worship and a refuge for the small local community, within its four chambers, one above the other, from Viking raiders. It remains mostly as it was built except for battlements added about 1450 and a clock around 1650. Its thousandth anniversary was celebrated with noteworthy heartiness and pride in 1970.

As for William's second objective of obtaining domestic support and participation, he does not seem to have met many difficulties once he had kindled the avarice of his knights and other fighting men, and had dulled any pangs of conscience they might have had by quoting Pope Alexander's blessing upon his invasion-crusade. William achieved his purpose by calling assemblies of his magnates at Lillebonne, Bonneville-sur-Toques and other centres within his Duchy at which men agreed to join and serve him on promises of splendid rewards to come, according to the contributions they made, in the form of English lands and treasure which would fall into Norman hands once Harold had been mastered. In June, 1066, William used the occasion of the dedication of Mathilda's church of the Holy Trinity at Caen to stir more secular and ecclesiastical fervour for his enterprise through addresses and informal talks with his lords and prelates gathered there. The Norman archives show that the assembly at Lillebonne was probably the biggest and most decisive of all the meetings; it was also the most impressive, being held in the great hall of a fortress which had seen history made since Roman times, when Lillebonne was known as Juliobona, and was to stand for several centuries after the eleventh as a monument to the talents of early Norman designers and builders.

William also smoothly gained his third objective of making the Duchy secure while he was away. He conferred powers of attorney on his diminutive Mathilda and appointed viceroys to serve her while she ruled in his stead. Among these were the elderly Roger de Beaumont, who was later to be rewarded with the earldom of Leicester, and Hugh D'Avranches, who became Earl of Chester. As for the succession, William named his son Robert, then aged about fourteen, as his heir and commanded his principal barons to swear to recognize Robert as such.

If William could have foreseen the trouble which this vain, extravagant and feather-brained sprig was to cause him in his declining years he might have thought hard about nominating him in 1066, although William's behaviour towards Robert throughout their association suggests strikingly that, for all his sternness and resolution as a soldier and a statesman, he was a weak and doting parent. The son provoked his first dangerous breach with his father in 1077, when William was approaching 50 years of age, but one feels there must have been much earlier unrecorded friction. Spurred on by flattering companions, Robert demanded in 1077 that his father should yield to him control of Normandy and Maine. When William asked for time to consider the demand, Robert stupidly tried to enforce it peremptorily by attacking Rouen. William's loyal commanders and men beat him off, and Robert and his companions fled in disarray out of the Duchy. But Robert had not yet finished tormenting his father. He went into an alliance with the King of France and raised a second rebellion. The ageing William confronted him in January 1079 at Gerberoi, where Robert was strongly placed with his French, Breton and other allies in a castle. William besieged the castle but failed to take it and during a sortie by the defenders William had the humiliation of being unhorsed and then wounded in the hand by his own son. This was one of the few defeats ever suffered by William and it was certainly the worst. He might very well have been killed at Gerberoi had not an Englishman, Toki of Wallingford sacrificed his own life for William. Toki rushed up to the wounded William and set him upon a fresh horse so that he could get away from his attackers. Moments later Toki was struck and killed by a bolt from a rebel crossbow.

Fearing that one defeat might be followed by others, William made peace with his troublesome son. Surprisingly, they became reconciled and, even more surprisingly, William again named Robert as heir to the Duchy. But relations between them were still not good and even as William lay dying in 1087 Robert was again in revolt, but was not disinherited. Here indeed is an epic of astonishing paternal weakness and filial disdain and here too is disclosed one of the few frailties in William's character.

He showed none of this or any other kind of weakness in 1066. He seems to have been sharp and businesslike in his enrolment of his knights. Those agreeing to take part in the invasion were required to furnish men and ships as well as their own services and, although the surviving records are somewhat skimpy and occasionally unclear, it looks as if William exacted contributions in strict accordance with a graduated feudal scale according to the rank and importance of each participant, balanced by similarly exact potential rewards after victory. Mathilda joined the national effort by providing the flagship in which her husband was to lead the invasion fleet. The ship was named *Mora*, for some reason which has never emerged, and it is shown prominently in the Bayeux Tapestry with William at the tiller and a signal lantern surmounted by a cross at the masthead. An elaborately-carved figure blowing a horn and carrying a miniature lance and a gonfanon, or war pennant, is seen just behind and above William to confirm that this in fact is the flagship and the man guiding it the leader of the expedition. The *Mora* and all the other ships built by William's carpenters and shipwrights at various ports up and down the coast of Normandy were being sailed by the beginning of May to an assembly point at the mouth of the river Dives, 14 miles north-east of Caen and about 100 miles due south of the coast of Sussex. The assemblage of ships, warriors, horses, stores and equipment is estimated to have taken two months.

Tostig Rouses Support

On the other side of the Channel there had been many developments. Tostig was at the heart of most of them, always the irritant but more and more often now the desperate loser. Edwin and Morcar gave him one of his worst setbacks. Reacting as Harold had foreseen to a threat to their domains by an old enemy who had been ousted from Northumbria to make way for Morcar only two years earlier, they mobilized strongly against him and came upon him at some point inland from the long, flat coast of north Lincolnshire towards the end of May. They appear to have been able to take him by surprise, for he was ingloriously routed. He lost many of his men in battle and, as he and the survivors fled to their ships, hundreds of those whom he had forced into his service during earlier raids took this prime opportunity to desert him. He had only 12 ships left out of his original 60. In these he and the remnants of his once respectable army sailed again northwards. It is unclear whether Tostig had by this time encountered his accidental ally Copsi, but he probably had and so Copsi had shared in the debacle.

In extremity, having shot his bolt with small profit to himself, Tostig made for Scotland to seek sanctuary from King Malcolm, his blood brother. Theirs was an opportunistic partnership. They had gone through the rite of swearing loyalty to each other in 1059 when Tostig had formally escorted Malcolm southwards on a state visit to the court of Edward the Confessor, but, as with so many of today's national statesmen and leaders, they kept to the terms of the bond only when it suited them. Only two years after it had been sworn Malcolm took ruffianly advantage of Tostig's temporary absence from home. Tostig was sent by King Edward to accompany the newly-appointed Archbishop of York, Aldred, to Rome so that he could ceremonially receive his *pallium*, or symbol of office, from the Pope. The story of what happened while he was away is told by a reputable northern chronicler, Simeon of Durham. Malcolm invaded Tostig's lands in Northumbria and looted several areas of it, including the historic abbey of St Cuthbert on the island of Lindisfarne (Holy Island), two miles off the coast. This was the second time Lindisfarne had been ravaged by pillagers; in 793 it had been the first place in all England to have been attacked by Vikings. The abbey which Malcolm looted had been founded by Lindisfarne's sixth bishop, Cuthbert, and he had been buried there for many decades, until in threatening times his body was taken away for safety, first to Chester-le-Street and then to Durham.

Now in 1066 the two blood brothers allowed bygones to be forgiven and forgotten. Malcolm received Tostig and his bruised warriors into his castle at Dunfermline, and the pair proceeded to work out what profit they could gain together from the harassed kingdom of England to the south. Malcolm wanted territory and power and Tostig still wanted vengeance upon Harold. Dunfermline is 14 miles north-west of Edinburgh and was for several centuries a royal Scottish residence. Dunfermline Castle is also the resting-place of the bones of the renowned Robert the Bruce. Appropriately to our story, the city figures in a well-known Scottish ballad which contains the lines :

> The King sits in Dunfermline Town
> Drinking the blude-red wine.

It is not hard to picture King Malcolm and his possessed guest Tostig sitting at the blude-red wine as they plotted and bargained during the high summer of 1066. . . .

By this time something had obviously disrupted the partnership between Tostig and Duke William. William may now have concluded from Tostig's grim experience in Lincolnshire that his value as an ally had ended. Tostig on his part may have decided that, judging by the strength of Harold's defences and the savage handling which Edwin and Morcar had given him, William had little or no chance of making a successful descent upon England from across the Channel and that consequently he was not worth Tostig's continued support.

Several theories offer themselves as alternative explanations for Tostig's swing to the north after his defeat in Lincoln. He may simply have decided that Malcolm offered the best available sanctuary, but this is unlikely since he could more easily have turned south and gone back to Flanders. He may have worked out that the best opportunity to topple Harold lay in an invasion from the north, upon wild English territory which was far less thickly populated and much harder to defend than the south. Or he may have also decided to double-cross William; having trailed his coat in the south and thereby drawn all Harold's reserves into that region to prepare to repel William, he now hoped to find partners such as Malcolm in a swift thrust from Scotland which would forestall William and probably turn out to be almost unopposed by Harold. In view of what happened in the late summer this last theory would seem the valid one.

Tostig's whole career testifies to his impetuous, treacherous and cruel nature, and it appears that he was envious of his elder brother, Harold, even before the episode which ended his tenure of the earldom of Northumbria. Henry, Archbishop of Huntingdon, in a chronicle written early in the twelfth century, relates an act said to have been committed by Tostig which reflects this jealousy as well as his awful ferocity. It is described so circumstantially that it must have had some foundation in truth. It happened in 1065 during one of Tostig's periods of high uncontrollability just before he was banished from Northumbria, and may well have been one of the reasons why King Edward and Harold agreed to his banishment. The Archbishop says that one day at Windsor, Tostig and Harold were with the King and as they talked together Harold proffered a cup of wine or other refreshment to Edward. A sudden and irrational fury seized Tostig at this seeming evidence of Harold's closeness to the King. He turned upon his brother, tugging at his hair. There was a scuffle which was broken up before any serious harm was done, but the King was so incensed by Tostig's mad onslaught that he ordered Tostig permanently from his court. Tostig thereupon rode in even greater fury to Hereford, where Harold had a manor at which his servants were making ready to receive and entertain the King. Tostig and his men hacked off the heads, arms and legs of some of the servants and stuffed them into containers of wine and ale. They then rode off, Tostig leaving a message for his brother and the King to the effect that since he knew they were going to have a great feast together he had supplied them with plenty of salted meats to go with their other food.

The story could be an exaggerated version of what happened. More important, however, is the fact that a virtually contemporary chronicler, and one of high clerical rank, should have written it at all. It provides some quite valuable confirmation of Tostig's character and reputation – that he was probably unbalanced, savage, and had an uncontrollable temper. If he had been otherwise, the Archbishop of Huntingdon would surely have dismissed the story as impossible and not included it in his chronicles. These are well-ordered and apparently accurate on the whole.

Further evidence of Tostig's repellent character comes from the Orkneyinga Saga (a chronicle of events in the north which is notable for its unequivocal descriptions of its heroes and villains): 'Tostig was a tall man and a strong, scowling-browed one, a great man for words and the most warlike of men; he did not have many friends.'

The outcome of discussions between Tostig and Malcolm in the halls of Dunfermline Castle was that besides coming to an agreement between themselves, they turned to a new ally who was also a formidable challenger for the throne of England – Harald Hardrada, King of Norway. It fitted their designs that they should go to him. Neither Malcolm nor Tostig wanted England for himself because each knew he could not possibly make himself acceptable to the people. But Harald Hardrada, a Viking enjoying family and friendly links with the country, could probably do so, and in partnership with him Malcolm and Tostig would have an excellent chance of joining in the overthrow of Harold and sharing the consequent booty of lands and power.

Contemporary reporters in England assumed, in the absence of information to the contrary, that Tostig stayed with Malcolm for the rest of the summer until the last days of September when, as we shall see, he emerged to start his final, fatal venture against his brother. This assumption would help to explain why the intrusion of Harald Hardrada into the drama of 1066 apparently came as such a surprise to the English. An analysis of events during the rest of the year points strongly to the probability that after Tostig and Malcolm had decided on a plan of action, Tostig sailed off from Scotland on a secret visit to Hardrada to propose the terms of the triangular partnership they had in mind. That Tostig went all the way to Norway to interview Hardrada is stated categorically by some Norwegian chroniclers. They say that the pair met at Viken and one poetical reporter, Snorri Sturlasen, the Icelandic bard whose evocative powers exceed those of the most fluent of Norman scribes, even ventures to paraphrase the conversation between the two. We may prudently accept the fact of the meeting, but not Snorri's embellishments. The outlines of the bargain proposed by Tostig were as follows. Hardrada would mobilize in the Orkneys and when he sailed south from there he would make for an intermediate base, where he would receive supplies and reinforcements from Malcolm. Tostig would join him at some agreed point so that they could make a combined invasion of northern England. The odds were strongly in their favour that they could secure a vast stretch of territory from which neither William nor Harold, whichever one had survived an encounter between them, could really hope to dislodge them. Tostig would be rewarded with the return of his lost earldom of Northumbria or whatever else he chose as an equivalent; Malcolm would get a free hand to absorb territory south of his constricted kingdom around the Firth of Forth; and Hardrada would fulfil a dream by adding at least a major part of England to his royal possessions.

Hardrada agreed to the proposition. How could he possibly refuse it? He was a restless adventurer, ever ready for aggressive action. He was also one of the most celebrated fighting men of his times and outsize in both character and physique. He must have been an unforgettable figure to anybody who encountered him either as friend or enemy. His hair was light blond and he had long blond moustaches. One eyebrow was permanently higher than the other. His hands and feet were large but well-proportioned and in accord with his great height of over seven feet. Writing from living memory of Hardrada, Snorri Sturlasen gives a concise description of his character: 'He was inordinately greedy for power and of valuable possessions of all kinds. But all who went campaigning with him and were with him in battle agree that whenever he was in great danger and everything depended on a quick decision he almost always hit upon a plan which in the event was seen by everybody to have been the one most likely to succeed.' His descriptive name, Hardrada, indicated his redoubtable personality. In strict translation it meant 'hard counsel'; in modern terms it may well be rendered as 'tough guy'. And that is what he was – a man who in his long life as a warrior had been a military terror in Africa, Sicily, Greece, Byzantium and Scandinavia, and was now ready to become the conqueror of England. At the age of 51, Hardrada was about the most experienced warrior chief in the western world. But he was physically well past his prime and the prospect of having the younger Tostig, still in his early forties, as an ally and sub-commander on the coming field of battle must have appealed to him, especially since Tostig was a brave and skilled fighter for all his faults. Hardrada's luck was to fail him at last this year and he was not destined to leave a permanent and decisive mark upon history. He was in fact one of history's great also-rans – a man who would be remembered for the strength of his arm and for his fabled deeds on the battlefield, deeds glowingly and of course exaggeratedly recounted by his bards, but of no real account in the moulding of the world to come after him. His one contribution to the outcome of the Conquest was similar to Tostig's – the fatal weakening of King Harold before William attacked him. Neither Hardrada nor Tostig was to survive to ponder the importance of his role.

Hardrada found a justification for an invasion of England by arguing that he had some claim to the throne of that country by virtue of a bargain made years earlier between him and King Harthacanute (1040–1042). It was enough to justify an offensive by a warrior of his self-confidence and ambition. There was also the lure of toppling King Harold Godwinson and forestalling Duke William in the process.

4

A Setback for the Duke

As William superintended the assembly of his mixed forces and his
fleet at the mouth of the River Dives, he could not be likened to a
monarch building a national army dedicated to the achievement
of a national purpose. He was, as the late Sir Charles Oman aptly
described him, 'rather the managing director of a great joint-stock
company for the conquest of England'. He did have that papal
blessing to provide an aura of moral justification for his invasion,
but in reality it was a coolly-planned aggression, for which William
was furnishing the impetus, organization and the leadership, while
his Norman and foreign lieutenants were contributing their quotas
of boats, arms, horses and fighting men, risking their own lives in
return for loot if they survived.

Men were perfectly willing to do this in the eleventh century.
They did not put such high value on life as we, more favoured
and with far more to lose in the enjoyments of existence, are prone
to do. But one assurance they did demand – that they were not
risking eternal damnation by joining William in his attack upon
Harold and England. This explains why William had gone to such
pains to obtain the Pope's approval and why the absolution it
implied was so disproportionately powerful a tool for recruitment.
In the last 500 years of its phenomenal germination and growth
in western Europe, Christianity had inspired revolutionary changes
in men's attitudes. One of the most effective of these changes
arose from Christianity's promise of life after death. It had
banished man's fears not of death itself but of the awful blankness
and nullity which followed it and against which he had thought he
could do nothing.

The heathen fears which Christianity had removed were elo-
quently summarized by Sir Arthur Bryant, the historian, in his
Makers of the Realm in 1953: 'They feared death and the un-

predictable forces of nature and the mysterious powers – demon and monster, giant and ghoul – with which they identified them. They feared the wild passions of human nature that unloosed so many disasters upon the world. And, though they faced their fears manfully, they did not believe that man in the end could master his fate or that anything could save him from his terrible dilemma and the annihilation that awaited him.'*

Now men did not necessarily have to face that frightening oblivion. Provided a man did not offend God, or provided he undertook a prescribed penance if he did (we have already noted how William and Mathilda compensated for the offence implied in their marriage, and we shall later come across more instances of the purchase of absolution), he need not fear the transition into death, for he would enjoy God's protection in the hereafter. If the Pope said that by invading England and conquering it, men were serving a holy purpose, they would not shrink from risking death to fulfil it, particularly as there could be great profit therein if all went well. Many of them would without doubt comfort themselves, as soldiers have done throughout the centuries, with the assurance that it would almost certainly be the other fellow who would be killed anyway. Soothed, then, by the principles and the hopes for the hereafter offered by the new faith of Christianity, men volunteered in profusion to serve under William. They surged into Normandy from almost all the provinces and duchies of northern Europe; some even came from Italy and as far south as Sicily.

William's carpenters and the artisan-soldiers in his army built hundreds of ships in the ports along the Norman coast and when these were finished they were all sailed towards the assembly areas at the Dives estuary. A modern concensus puts their number at about 700. They were of various sizes and types but they were all built comparatively lightly, to survive only a one-way trip across the Channel. There appear, however, to have been more boats of one particular kind than any other. These had one small steering oar but did not have rowing oars which would have taken up space needed for fighting men. They also had large sheet sails which have been estimated as giving them a maximum speed of about four knots in ideal conditions. They were between 40 and 50 feet long, took about four feet of water, and were open-decked and very broad in

* See Appendix B, p. 193.

the beam. They could not operate to windward because of their primitive equipment and they had to have a favourable wind to make any kind of headway. This limitation was one of the most important single factors in the timing of the invasion and consequently in the race for the prize of England between William and Hardrada. Lack of a fair wind held up William for several precious weeks, but the delay had the compensating decisive effect, as will become clear, of enabling him to make an unopposed crossing of the Channel and an unopposed landing upon the English shore.

In assembling a fleet composed mostly of such frail craft William was plainly staking everything upon victory. He foresaw that there would be no chance whatever of his force being able to make a return trip in case of defeat and he therefore wasted neither time nor effort in encumbering his ships with equipment and modifications which could never be used. He was being characteristically realistic. He knew that in the event of defeat in an open field battle the Normans, including unhorsed knights in heavy armour, would be under close attack right to the water's edge as they retreated. Even if some of them did manage to climb aboard a ship, what good would that do them? The chances of their then being able to hoist sail and make off before a favourable wind were virtually non-existent. No, if Harold routed William in the field it would have to be a case of every Norman for himself. The likeliest outcome would be that his men would scatter and seek to elude their pursuing victors by disappearing in twos and threes into the thinly-occupied countryside and then try to survive by whatever means they could find. Their best prospect would be to try and reach some of the many Normans who lived in England, for these would readily give the beaten fugitives succour and shelter and might even help them to promote a re-grouping and subsequent second attempt to conquer England by a land campaign alone.

William's task of enrolling, assembling and equipping his amphibious invasion force was a heavy one, and anybody with knowledge of military problems and techniques will not hesitate to applaud his effort in achieving it. It was nothing like so complicated, of course, as later similar efforts were to become as men found more and more effective and discreditable ways of assaulting and killing each other. William's true claim to recognition may rest more properly not on the magnitude of what he did but on having accomplished it so thoroughly, practically and, apparently, so quickly. One of his big advantages over succeeding seaborne commanders was that the practice of warfare in his time was still comparatively simple, not having changed in any important respects for several centuries. The only developments which were beginning to add to the preoccupations of a commander in his day were the growing use of the mounted warrior in Europe and the accompanying increase in the weightiness and intricacy of armour. Apart from these not yet unmanageable complications, a warrior's needs in offence and defence were still few. The only projectile, apart from the short-range spear and javelin and the stone lobbed at an oncoming enemy by sling or strong right arm, was the arrow, and soldiers had had to contend with that menace for many centuries. The bow as a weapon in war and in animal hunting is estimated by archeologists and historians to be between 30,000 and 40,000 years old. It is interesting that it appears to have been discovered and developed independently in those early times by men who could not possibly have had any contact or even have known of each other's existence on the planet. Wooden bows dating from the Stone Age have been found in western Europe and elsewhere, as have stone arrowheads.

For the rest, fighting was still hand to hand and the assets a warrior needed above all others were brute strength, co-ordination and quick reflexes, and reliable comrades to back him up in any sudden emergency. The weapons of 1066 most commonly used were the bow, spear and axe. While the havoc they caused was physically just as revolting as the later cannon, tank, machine gun, rifle, bomb and torpedo, their scope was very limited and they did not call for the array of human and technological supports needed by their successors. The only bothersome element in William's amphibious force was his cavalry – but the knights, squires and horses upon which he had to spend so much thought and attention as they gathered with him for the coming voyage from the mouth of the Dives, were to repay him handsomely on the field at Hastings.

Considering all the evidence available today it seems likely that William had between 3,000 and 4,000 knights and other mounted troops in his army. The cavalry was the elite, and in assembling and training this company of armed and armoured horsemen for use as a flying charge to cut a way through enemy infantry and then hack down beaten and fleeing men, William was following a growing practice among continental commanders. The only western nation which still fought only on foot was the English. Warriors of this race would usually ride their horses, or more accurately their ponies, to a battlefield. Then they would dismount and form a solid line several ranks deep behind a wall of shields. As long as this double barrier held firm, enemy foot soldiers and cavalry alike would charge in vain until both man and horse were exhausted and could themselves be pursued and cut down as they staggered away.

There is only one recorded instance of English warriors fighting on horseback, and it was obviously a pitiful failure. The Anglo-Saxon Chronicle describes an encounter at Hereford in 1035 between a combined Irish-Welsh army under an outlawed earl, Alfgar, and a big force of levies commanded by earl Ralph of Herefordshire (a nephew of Edward the Confessor): 'before a spear was thrown the English fled because they had been made to fight on horseback; many of them were slain, about four hundred or perhaps five, but none of their opponents.' It would seem that even in those days the islanders were obstinate, dedicated aherents of tradition and the *status quo ante*, worthy forefathers of those who until 1970 persisted in the confusing use of their monetary symbols of pounds, shillings and pence, and continued for long after that to ride and drive on the left-hand side of the road when most of the remainder of the world's peoples did the opposite. They regarded with suspicion the inevitable move into the European Common Market, and one out of every two of them was still verbally resisting it even after it had happened in 1973.

William's quartermasters, paymasters, victuallers, police and other ancillary professionals kept no permanent records of how they supplied and controlled the invasion force while it waited to sail. It was the most agreeable season of the year, the equivalent of the modern summer holiday period. The air of Normandy would be warm and soothing. The unpolluted sea was there to tempt the bather and the fisherman. Days were long and existence was a simple matter of eating, sleeping and enjoying oneself. A man could do as he wished with far more hours of leisure than are available today. We may presume that some of William's men would use them quietly and profitably, but we shall be wiser to believe that most of the waiting warriors squandered their time in the traditional pleasures of wine, women and song (plus a few others) and inevitably got into mischief and trouble. The only surviving mention of what

must have been a lively summer by the sea is from William of
Poitiers and, as so often, he is sickeningly fulsome towards William's
interests and in most respects so deliberately misleading as to be
useless. Paying the customary tribute to William, he writes: 'Such
was his moderation and prudence that he utterly forbade pillage,
and provided for fifty thousand soldiers [!] at his own cost for a
whole month while contrary winds delayed them at the mouth of
the Dives. He made generous provision both for his own knights
and those from other parts, but he did not allow any of them to take
their sustenance by force. The flocks and herds of the peasantry
pastured unharmed throughout the province. The crops waited
undisturbed for the sickle without being trampled by the pride of
the knights or ravaged by the greed of the plunderers. A weak and
unarmed man, watching the swarm of soldiers without fear, might
follow his horse singing wherever he would.' What an idyll! What
balderdash!

The much more likely truth is that William and his administrators were faced with as much as they could manage in coping
with some 12,000 (not 50,000!) high-spirited and mettlesome men,
many of whom turned to roystering, marauding and 'other Vices
which effeminate men's minds', as Milton put it pregnantly, many
years later. Throughout history armies of arrayed but inactive
men have been notoriously licentious and troublesome, only slightly
less so than armies of occupation. There is no reason to suppose that
William's waiting horde was an exception. We can only assume
that William of Poitier's incredible passage was prompted by the
need he felt to hide the ugly truth and at the same time protect his
master's reputation before history. One fact may be taken as certain.
William was a stern commander and he had already shown that he
knew how to handle men, friends or enemies. He would punish
flagrant offenders without mercy as an example to the rest of his
men.

As a militarist with a strong Viking heritage and as a ruler with
a coastline of his own to control, stretching some 250 miles from
one end of his Duchy at Mont St Michel in the west to Le Tréport
in the east, William understood and respected the sea. He knew
a good deal about the dangers contained in its unpredictable
vagaries and tantrums. (For all his knowledge and his innate
caution, it was to play a costly trick upon him before long.) He
knew that no matter what alternative plans he made and what

precautions he took, he could be upset by one of those familiar sudden changes in Channel conditions. He also knew that although the Channel was broad between Normandy and England and offered plenty of room for manoeuvre because it was so empty of shipping, he could not count upon making either an unobserved or unopposed crossing or an unopposed landing in Sussex. But he could reasonably expect that enough of his ships would survive a slow-moving sea battle to make a landing still possible, and it was doubtful if Harold, whom he knew to be in a weak political position in England, could muster enough troops to beat off invaders who were concentrated at one particular point along the coast. Although Harold's fleet lying off the coast of the Isle of Wight was big, it was also makeshift, hastily mobilized and manned for the most part by inexperienced sailors recruited from the villages, ports and settlements of southern and western England.

William, who was of course well-informed about the state of England, knew very well that Harold had had no permanent fleet at his disposal when he became king only a few months ago, for Edward the Confessor had long before (in 1050) disbanded the small flotilla of 16 warships which he had inherited from King Canute; and, incidentally, there had never been a standing army in England. Edward, no warrior king and a rarity in an era when most potentates were for ever leading their forces against an enemy, had been satisfied to rely on naval strength through an arrangement whereby the ports of Sandwich, Dover, Fordwich, Romney, and probably Hastings and Rye as well, agreed to furnish men and ships on demand in return for royal charters granting them special privileges. These towns alone could not possibly have supplied all the strength Harold needed in 1066, and it is a tribute to his determination that he was able to assemble a defensive fleet of unprecedented size from next to nothing and very rapidly. One factor in his favour was of course that the southern and western ports and communities from which he drew conscripts and volunteers were in his own former earldom of Wessex or in territory which had long been possessed by the House of Godwin, and they would therefore be the loyal sources, perhaps the only loyal sources in England, open to him.

This fleet, having no projectiles other than its seaman's bows and spears, would have to make a close physical interception to attempt and achieve its deterrent purpose, and there were tactics available to William to avoid damaging contact with it. He could, for example, take an evasive course with most of his fleet from the moment he and Harold's fleet sighted each other, leaving a strongly-armed rearguard of expendable ships to take the brunt of any assault while the bulk of the invasion force continued its course towards England. Or, if wind and weather and comparative speeds permitted, he could lead the whole of his invasion force away from Harold's pursuing vessels towards England or back to Normandy. Adjudging William's inclinations from all the known facts about his military career, we can probably assume that if at all possible he would head for England, for he was not the sort to retreat in the hope of fighting another day under better circumstances. After all, William's own Viking ancestors had been proving for generations that it was easy to get ashore along the thinly-populated coasts of the island and, even while he had been building his fleet, Tostig had been confirming the fact and at the same time showing that Harold probably did not have enough troops to resist and rout even a small invading force.

Tostig had been able to get ashore with even his minute striking force – but, significantly, he had not been able to stay there because Harold did have his Housecarls and auxiliaries whom he could despatch to smite those who made a lodgement; Tostig had usually not even waited to be attacked. So the big question which must have exercised William's mind while he waited at the Dives estuary for a favourable southerly or south-easterly wind was whether Harold would be strong enough to overcome the very powerful force which William hoped to land in Sussex. This was something which would be proved or disproved solely by battle.

William is estimated to have been ready to sail by the second week in August* but was then heavily delayed first by the long lack of a southerly wind, and then by mishaps caused again by the elements. But, everything considered, he was lucky in experiencing all his setbacks in the early phase of his adventure, when they could be digested and rectified without interference, and not, as did Harold, when he had been brought face to face with his enemies and was under many pressures.

---

* See Appendix C (p. 196) for on outline of the ingenious calculations whereby this date is reached.

The Fleet Sails

At last, the wind began to blow from the south one day in early September, and William decided to go. In doing so he had to rely almost entirely on his own judgement and luck. He had, of course, no skilled professionals with their sensitive instruments and their precise knowledge to give him guidance on what the weather might be for even 24 hours ahead – a precious advantage available to General Eisenhower in coming to a similar decision 878 years later. One imagines that William talked the matter over with his chief lieutenants but they knew no more than he about possibilities and probabilities concerning Channel weather, and a firm mind such as William's would be unlikely to be much swayed by what any of them advised. He would scarcely have been human, however, if he had not been influenced towards an affirmative by weeks of frustration caused not only by the stubborn absence of a southerly wind but also, probably, by experiencing several missed chances of setting sail, when the weather unexpectedly turned favourable just long enough to make the trip across the Channel.

What a stately sight William's 700 ships must have presented as they moved slowly, probably as dawn was breaking, out to sea from Normandy! If the Bayeux Tapestry is to be believed in this context, and it is our only authority, William's ships, made solely for this high adventure of invasion, were appropriately graceful and heroic-looking. The *Mora*, William's flagship, and other craft used only to carry warriors and knights were part-gondola and part-barge. Their bows reared vertically in the shape of the head of a sea-horse and their sterns curled upwards to give the effect of a beast's tail. Others which had been built for the transport of horses, bulky baggage, arms and stores were more severely practical but none the less picturesque in their way.

The Tapestry is impressively informative about the fleet in some particulars – showing, for example, that masts were made from sturdy but only rough-carpentered tree trunks – but is palpably inaccurate in others, perhaps because the artistic designers of the Tapestry wanted to make William's ships look as majestic as they could. They foreshortened some of the ships to get as many as possible into their panorama. But the estimate that most of them were some 50 feet long, less than half the size of the great sea-going 'double-ender' Viking ships used during the preceding two centuries, seems valid. It received some indirect but persuasive confirmation during the 1960s when five Viking ships which had been sunk to block the fairways of Roskilde Fiord, in Denmark, from attacks by Norwegian raiders between 1000 and 1050 were painstakingly recovered and remodelled from thousands of salvaged fragments. One of them had an uncanny likeness to the *Mora* as shown in the Tapestry. It was 54 feet long, 8 feet wide, 3 feet 6 inches high amidships and its prow and stern bore the motif of the sea-horse. Nobody can say what connection there was between this ship and its sister, the *Mora*, but it is noteworthy that both were built at about the same period.

In the Tapestry the *Mora* is shown carrying ten men, including William. The others were presumably his principal lieutenants, perhaps including Bishop Odo, and his bodyguard. Most of the other ships are seen carrying light loads. In some panels men and horses are travelling together – eight men and their eight horses in one ship and nine of each in another. Elsewhere men are travelling without horses, and vice versa. In one ship 14 men are shown, but in another only three horses resting comfortably amidships with only two attendants, one apparently serving as lookout in the prow and the other at the steering oar aft. How factual these cameos are is impossible to tell, but it should be remembered that the designers and executants of the Tapestry were probably not sea-going people at all and that the purpose of the Tapestry was propagandistic as well as artistic.

William's ill-luck began not long after he had put out to sea. He had left the Dives at or soon after dawn for strictly practical reasons. At his estimated speed of four knots he had to allow a full 24 hours for the crossing to Pevensey, and he would obviously wish to make the last quarter or one-third of the journey in darkness, since this would be the period of greatest danger of interception by Harold's warships lurking off the Isle of Wight. But at some point after the Norman fleet put out to sea – nobody can know exactly when, for no precise account was ever allowed to be given – a storm struck the straggling fleet.

William was evidently taking an indirect course to England, hugging his own coastline as he sailed north-east towards Dieppe and Le Tréport before swinging due north for the comparatively brief dash of some 60 miles directly across-Channel to Pevensey. This is, incidentally, precisely the same kind of manoeuvre made by the

British and Belgian sea ferries plying between the English ports and Dunkirk and Ostend when the weather is uncertain. Although no hard evidence of any kind exists, an intelligent guess would be that the storm in 1066 struck William soon after he had ordered the change of course from east-south-east along the Norman coast to one of due north for Pevensey.

Some analysts of the Conquest doubt that William was ever hit by a storm and they make the plausible but unsupported assumption that he always intended to divide his cross-Channel trip into two stages. But adequate grounds for believing that this was not so are provided by the writings of the inevitable William of Poitiers who seems to have been the only Norman scribe permitted to hint, in his own devious and dissembling fashion, at the highly damaging setback which the weather inflicted upon William. He is convincing in spite of his distortions. He writes : 'The whole fleet most carefully equipped had for long waited for a south wind at the mouth of the Dives and in the neighbouring ports, but now by a west wind it was driven thence towards the harbour of St Valery. But the prince, daunted neither by the delay nor the contrary winds, nor by the loss of ships, nor even the craven flight of many who broke faith with him, commended himself with prayers and gifts and vows to the protection of Heaven. In his adversity he prudently concealed his lack of supplies by increasing the daily rations and, as far as he could, he caused those who had perished in the storm to be secretly buried.'

This singular passage in the chronicler's narrative is worth closer scrutiny. In the usual manner of the practised propagandist he discloses part of the truth in a show of mock frankness, hoping that by so doing he will successfully mask the darker facts. He first implies that the fleet was merely 'driven' by a west wind towards St Valery, but then he slips in references to 'the loss of ships' and the 'craven flight' of frightened deserters, and finally he mentions the secret burial of those who 'had perished in the storm'. It is quite clear if we read between the lines that the invasion fleet was very severely mauled by an unexpected Channel storm and might have been permanently dispersed but for William's innate resolution and quality of leadership. Further, he must have been on a course very close to his coast, since the bodies of many of his drowned men were apparently quickly washed ashore and secretly buried soon afterwards. Finally, there is considerable justification for believing that this episode forms one of those stifled stories which mark history, particularly military history, throughout the ages. The censor is not a modern phenomenon. Not one word or hint of the storm appears in the Bayeux Tapestry, not a word in the writings of any other chroniclers but William's propagandist who could be relied upon to gloss expertly over the real facts.

The damaged and depleted striking force of ships, men, horses, stores must have been a sorry sight, in depressing contrast to its aspect when it left Normandy, as it crawled into the harbours and inlets of the coast in the area of St Valery. This was not Norman territory since it lay a few miles east of the border of William's Duchy, but it was friendly country and offered him sure sanctuary. It was in fact part of a friendly coast of several hundred miles stretching from Brittany to what is now Belgium. What did not actually belong to William was possessed by allies or by sworn vassals. He therefore was certain of succour no matter where he might have to make a forced landfall after leaving Normandy. St Valery was in country belonging to the same Guy de Ponthieu, William's vassal who, according to the Bayeux Tapestry, had arrested Harold in unclear circumstances about two years earlier. Here William could take whatever time he needed for recovery and replacement. The worst sufferers during the storm must have been the horses: standing or lying in the cramped transports they would have been virtually helpless as the boats tossed and whipped about in the tempest, and their attendants would be in no state to do much more than preserve themselves, too seasick to tend the horses. Nothing exact is known about the extent of the damage caused to the invasion fleet, but we have evidence that William eventually lay in St Valery for 15 days; that is to say, probably from 12–13 September until 27 September, when he at last sailed for Pevensey.

Some historians and analysts have, surprisingly in all the circumstances, cast doubt on the story that William was driven ashore at St Valery against his will. They have preferred to believe that William sailed from the Dives to St Valery by intent, that the storm, if it ever happened, was merely an incident during the planned trip and that, once again, William of Poitiers elaborated on it only to laud and magnify the name of his earthly patron. This interpretation is presumably founded on a theory that William would find it practical and to his advantage to make the voyage to England in two stages because by sailing at ease north-eastwards to St Valery in the protected and sheltered waters close to his coast he would thereby be narrowing the gap across the Channel between him and England to one of only some 60 miles and would also be much further from the Isle of Wight and Harold's fleet than a more direct crossing from the Dives would have entailed.

The theory certainly suits the facts of what actually happened, to William's eventual advantage, but it weakens under scrutiny. For one thing, William of Poitiers, the official mouthpiece, would almost certainly not have included in his version of the storm the revealing phrases about the loss of ships, the desertions and the secret burials of the storm's victims if nothing of any consequence had really happened. Further, an expert commander such as Duke William would not be likely to squander a long-awaited opportunity to sail from Normandy before a suitable wind on such a half-measure as a trip along his coast to another port only indirectly on the way to his objective at Pevensey. He would be much more inclined to make his invasion in one operation. Having gone through the complicated and tiresome business of getting everybody and every-thing aboard his ships he would not relish having to unload them again at St Valery and repeat the process all over again, subject all the while to the caprices and dangers of the Channel weather. Surely if he had intended to cross from St Valery from the beginning he would have sent all his knights and their horses and as much of his stores as possible there by land from the assembly point at the Dives, leaving only lightly-loaded and lightly-manned craft to make the coastal sea trip. There would be no point, and indeed there would be much discomfort and avoidable risk, in sending the whole force by sea to St Valery when most of it could get there comfortably in easy stages and in complete safety by land.

At about the same period of the year in 1940, Adolf Hitler moved *his* invasion boats out of contention from a stretch of the French coast which included St Valery – and he did it by sending his would-be invasion troops and their equipment out of danger by land; he sent only their unladen barges by sea.* All points considered,

---

* The author was stationed at Dover in September, 1940, as a correspondent assigned to report the German invasion of England if it should happen. One remarkably clear day late in the month he saw through binoculars a

it seems to be as certain as anything can be shown to be, after such a long span of time, that William reacted boldly to his opportunity when it presented itself in early August. Here at last was a favourable wind which, with luck, might last long enough for him to get to Pevensey in one move. It seems highly probable that he ordered everybody aboard, everything loaded and set off at last. He was taking a justifiable risk and it is not at all to his discredit that he temporarily lost the gamble.

There is an alternative theory. It has the attraction of fitting both Channel weather conditions and our estimate of William's calculating temperament. In other words, it implies the kind of manoeuvre such a man would make and explains how he came unluckily to be trapped by the storm with all his ships at sea. According to this theory (which the author now offers as a highly likely explanation of what happened), he sailed out from the Dives with two possible and alternative plans in his mind. He would take a north-easterly course close to his own shoreline for some hours and then, if wind and weather held good, veer north and head directly for Pevensey. But if it seemed that the wind was either changing or dropping or that the weather as a whole looked uncertain and unlikely to remain favourable long enough to give his fleet a quick cross-Channel passage, he would turn south-east (or whatever direction a changing wind indicated) towards his own coast only a few miles away, to take shelter in a port or even a series of inlets until the south wind came back. If this second alternative were forced upon him he would still have improved his tactical position by shortening the distance and dangers of the voyage to England in the open Channel, since he would have been advancing closer to his target with every hour at sea from the Dives.

In the event, the weather unexpectedly showed its mastery over man and his calculations. The storm came upon William too suddenly for him to do anything to cope with it, in one of those surprising changes for which conditions in the English Channel are

---

string of German invasion barges travelling slowly eastwards between Boulogne and Calais, some 20 miles across the Channel from the Shakespeare Cliff.

It later became known that the craft were on the move because Hitler had decided, finally, to abandon his proposed invasion and was sending the unladen barges beyond Calais to more remote havens in Belgium and Holland so that they should no longer attract the destructive attention of the Royal Air Force to the already severely battered Channel ports in France.

notorious. It drove his ships, helpless because of their burden and their primitive equipment, like leaves in an autumn wind and there was nothing for a man to do but to hope to survive until the shore was reached – in the area of St Valery.

Miraculously, the delay imposed upon him by the storm worked almost supernaturally to his eventual advantage. The sequence of developments on both sides of the Channel during September makes one wonder if some mysterious force determining man's destiny was not working tortuously but inexorably in favour of the man from Normandy and against the man from Wessex.

Unlucky Defender

Harold's fleet and his militia, or fyrd, had been fully mobilized since early July. This was before William could reasonably be expected to be ready to invade, but, as the prospective defender, Harold simply had to be ready in good time to meet his enemy. July was by no means too early for a threatened king to call his men together from the shires and scattered settlements of southern England, so that they could become known to each other and could be trained for the severe task of defence which surely lay ahead. William had made repeated declarations from January onwards that he was going to wrest his promised throne from the usurper, and these were supported by the plausible reports which reached Harold of William's methodical preparations for a Channel crossing. As the Anglo-Saxon Chronicle recorded, he had been reliably informed that Duke William meant to come to England and annex the country.

But William did not come as week after week of the summer slipped by. One delaying factor after another was holding him in check – the necessity to build a force big enough to ensure victory, a month of adverse and doubtful weather, and finally the storm in the Channel. But if that storm had not held up William beyond 8 September, if he had been able to cross to England before that date, he would have run the risk of interception by sea from the Isle of Wight as well as early resistance on land by Harold's defenders at Pevensey. There is no doubt whatever that 8 September is the crucial date on which the fortunes of the two contestants in 1066 were drastically altered, to William's great advantage. This was the day after which his success in making a firm lodgement was assured. Once again the Anglo-Saxon Chronicle tells the story. After describing Harold's mobilization by sea and land it states: 'When the Festival of the Nativity of St Mary [8 September] came, the men's provisions had run out, and nobody could keep them there any longer; they were therefore given permission to return home. Then the King rode up and the ships were sailed into London, but many were lost before they arrived.'

Harold's luck was out. His mobilization had turned out to be a disruptive and expensive waste of effort, and even when he had given way to overpowering pressures of reality by dispersing his fleet, the elements turned upon him and sank many of his precious ships before they could reach the sanctuary of the Thames. It is evident that neither Harold nor the country had the ability to keep a fleet and an army in being even semi-permanently. Although many of the arrangements concerning military service in pre-Conquest England are not known, it does seem that the king's power of conscription was limited. For example, except in extreme emergency he could muster an army only in the proportion of one warrior for every five hides of settled territory. This does not give us an unequivocal yardstick because the size of a hide as a unit of land measure appears to have varied from earldom to earldom – from 120 acres here to 30 or 40 acres there, according to a locality's value and fertility as well as to the local definition of a hide – but it does confirm that the more prosperous an area the more soldiers it had to provide. In many shires a man's term of service was limited to two months in a year or at a time, and this fact severely limited Harold's defensive capacity. Another factor implicit in the Chronicle's announcement of the demobilization on 8 September is that the resources of the Isle of Wight were not equal to sustaining 'the biggest fleet ever assembled by an English king' and that, similarly, the southern shires could not maintain for long the rations of the coastal guards quartered upon them in addition to feeding the local people.

A further factor would be the unsettlement among the soldiers and sailors which would grow with continued inactivity and the approach of autumn; they would become more and more uneasy knowing that they were being increasingly missed at home. The harvest was ripening and would soon have to be gathered and stored so that communities could live on, however primitively, and sheds and huts for the cattle had to be put into good repair against the coming winter. The help of every able-bodied man, and a warrior was certainly that, would be needed at home in the early autumn. Harold's men must have grown unsettled and uneasy as they asked themselves and each other: What good are we doing here waiting for an enemy who never comes?

Much can be read into the phrase in the Chronicle's account of the summer: 'Nobody could keep them there any longer. . . .' It is easy to imagine the pressures upon Harold. One must have been desertion.

So, as the days shortened and September fled by, the two principals in the drama of 1066 were temporarily at stalemate. Harold's England was as defenceless after 8 September as England was to be again in 1939 when threatened by another would-be invader. And William was, for a while, powerless to take advantage of this weakness because of adverse weather which, if he had ventured against it, would surely have taken as heavy a toll of his fleet as it took of Harold's. The only leading players whose fortunes seemed to be prospering in mid-September were Harald Hardrada and his ally, Tostig.

5

The Norwegian Pretender
Intervenes

Some 800 miles away to the north-east of St Valery and 300 miles across the North Sea from the Scottish mainland, Harald Hardrada's invasion fleet had been gathering during August in the Sulen Isles at the mouth of the Sognes Fiord, north of Bergen. It is estimated to have left there and headed due west on a favourable wind for the Shetland Isles about one month after Duke William had set off with *his* invasion fleet from the Dives estuary. The Shetlands, bleak and lonely fragments lapped by both the Atlantic and the North Sea, made a handy staging post for Harald Hardrada; they were more than half-way from Bergen to the Orkneys, which in their turn formed a second staging post on the northern doorstep of the land mass of Scotland. Both clusters of islands were Norwegian territory, under Hardrada's domination. They conveniently divided up the long distance from his homeland to his new target, England. His was to be an invasion on easy terms – until the final reckoning before the end of September.

Hardrada was in fact fulfilling a long-cherished idea in making this assault upon England. He had considered for many years that he had a title to it, as we have noted, and in 1058 he had given Edward the Confessor and Earl Harold (whom he had already perceived to be a rival contender for the succession) a reminder of his presence in the arena. He sent a Viking fleet under the command of his son, Magnus, to operate in the Irish Sea with the forces of Griffith of Wales. In one of those complex episodes in pre-Conquest England of which so few details are now known that it is quite impossible to comprehend them, Griffith was continuing his lifelong harassment of English authority by trying to secure the reinstatement of a banished nobleman, Alfgar, as Earl of Mercia. Griffith's activities offered Hardrada a useful opportunity to meddle in English affairs and to promote a campaign which might very well develop so as to give Magnus a chance to land on the western coast of Wales or England and stay there until Hardrada could join him and enlarge the landing into an assault against the whole kingdom. Magnus and Griffith succeeded in the limited objective of rein-stating Alfgar but they got no further. The English chroniclers dismissed this portentous episode in a few curt and impatient words – 'it is tedious to tell how it happened' – but the Irish diarists were much more revealing. One of them wrote in the Annals of Tigernach that a fleet 'led by the son of the King of the Scandinavians, along with the Foreigners of the Orkneys, and of the Hebrides, and of Dublin, came in order to take the Kingdom of England.' Then he added : 'But God permitted it not.'

Hardrada's effort in 1058 seems to have been more of a speculation than an organized invasion. But he was surely in earnest in 1066. The moment was more propitious for a move by him than it had been for many years. Edward the Confessor had been king, and quite firmly so, for 16 years in 1058 and few people in England would have relished or supported the onset of a foreign invader to oust him. But now a dubiously legal successor had been in power only shakily for nine months and was the most vulnerable monarch the country had had since Ethelred the Unready. Harald Hardrada would never again be offered such a providential opportunity to capture England, and he was in a position to grasp it.

How could Hardrada apparently prepare and carry out an invasion so much more quickly and easily than Duke William? The explanation lies of course in his superior military and tactical situation. As the ruler of a nation of Vikings, who for centuries had been as much at home afloat as on land, he had an abundant reserve of trained and seasoned sailors and soldiers; and almost every able-bodied Norwegian of the time was a willing and capable warrior and adventurer. Hardrada also had a powerful fleet stationed permanently at points along his coast. It was almost continuously in action or readiness. Less than three years earlier Hardrada had led 150 of his ships into a fierce sea battle lasting a day and a night against the fleet of Sweyn, King of Denmark. Harald had won that battle but it had still not gained him Denmark and had thereby perpetuated a strange career of outrageous but mostly profitless violence.

Harald's warships, most of which were kept permanently at readiness and available to him, were much bigger and far more effective fighting units than the expendable ones which William had built for the short one-way trip between Normandy and England. The backbone of Harald's fleet was the redoubtable Longship which Vikings had used for their piratical raids in northern latitudes for almost 300 years and which had been in particular a sore torment to England ever since the first sinister convoy of them appeared off Lindisfarne in 793. An average Longship was 80 feet long. It had a stout mast and a large square sail, and it was also fitted with between 10 and 20 crossbenches to accommodate between 20 and 40 oarsmen who could propel the narrow-beamed craft across the sea when the weather failed, or into and out of action at speed. Its full complement was approximately three times the number of oarsmen so that there were always 40 to 80 men ready for any emergency at sea or for an attack upon an enemy. The Longship did resemble William's smaller vessels in a few points. It was fitted with one small steering oar and it usually had some ornamental coloured carving, often of a dragon, rearing up from the prow. Obviously, it was a formidable fighting weapon in the hands of the cruel and fearless Scandinavian pirates and vandals.

Hardrada had one other advantage over William so far as speed of mobilization and mobility were concerned. He was not seeking to make history by carrying knights, horses and their armour and paraphernalia across the ocean in ships. In his land battles he had almost always fought on foot, and at the age of over 50 he was not contemplating making hazardous experiments. He calculated that he would be able to seize whatever number of horses he needed in England from peasants and farmers in the areas he conquered and occupied or even from well-disposed settlers of Viking descent whom he could expect to encounter in the Danelaw, a vast chunk of eastern and north-eastern England established in a treaty between King Alfred and the Danish invader Guthrum 176 years earlier, and also in the former independent kingdom of York, containing territory in which Hardrada proposed to operate during his invasion. York had been the seat of a line of local Scandinavian kings for many decades until Eric Bloodaxe, a Norwegian, was expelled by Anglo-Danes in 954. These various links between Scandinavia and England serve to emphasize that Hardrada was not a truly alien invader but one who could claim an association with the country he hoped to annex even if he did not have a serious claim to its throne.

Finally, Hardrada could thank Duke William himself for ensuring an easy and probably unopposed landing by the Norwegian host upon the shores of north-eastern England. The eyes of King Harold were turned in absorption towards the English Channel and all his defensive forces, or whatever remained of them after the enforced dispersal of so many reserves on 8 September, were being held in southern England to meet the expected coming of the Normans. It seems certain that nobody in any position of authority in England had any idea that Harald Hardrada was on his way. Hardrada, Tostig and Malcolm had prepared the blow secretly and at remarkable speed. There was really no time nor any means for King Harold to learn of it. Communications between England and Scotland by sea or by the vast, thinly-peopled and virtually roadless mass of Northumbria were scanty and haphazard. The first inkling anybody in northern England would have of the invasion would probably come when Hardrada appeared offshore, and it was likely that a fighting machine such as his would speed ahead of whatever stray travellers were abroad in those forbidding northern regions. Hardrada and Tostig could calculate that they would be able to put ashore without meeting resistance of any strength; they could also probably count on being able to establish themselves strongly before the regional forces of Earls Edwin and Morcar were mobilized against them. And Harald Hardrada, the confident conquering hero of so many mighty battles in the last half century, was a heavy favourite to defeat any militia which the earls could field against him.

Hardrada took with him as far as the Shetlands and Orkneys his wife, Ellisef, daughter of a Russian nobleman, and their daughters, Maria and Ingegerd. He also took with him one of his two sons, Olaf, a youth, leaving behind in Norway his elder son, Magnus, to serve as temporary ruler there in his stead. He also left behind one half of the able-bodied men in his kingdom to fight for Magnus if the need arose. Neither of these sons was Ellisef's. In the free-living fashion of the times in countries far from the supervision of Rome, Hardrada had 'married' a second wife, Thora, daughter of a Norwegian magnate named Thorberg Arneson, presumably because Ellisef had delivered only daughters to him and was now getting beyond the age when she could produce either son or daughter.

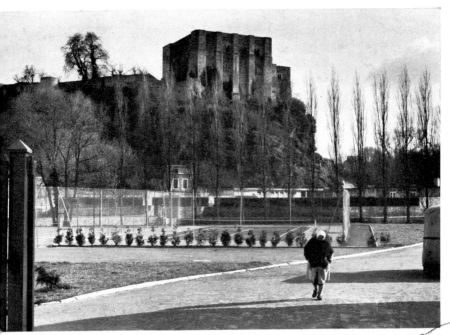

The massive castle built by William the Conqueror still dominates Falaise, his principal headquarters in his Duchy.

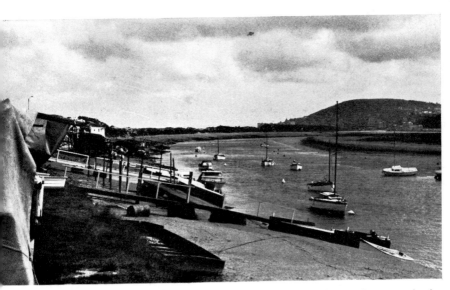

A yacht club flourishes today where the River Dives makes its final swing towards the Normandy coast. Here William's invasion fleet assembled in late summer, 1066.

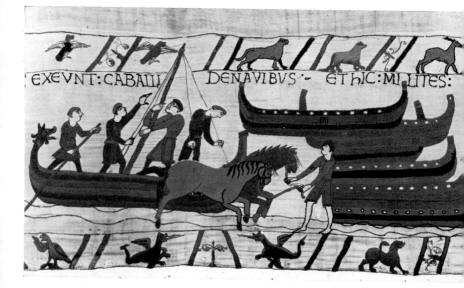

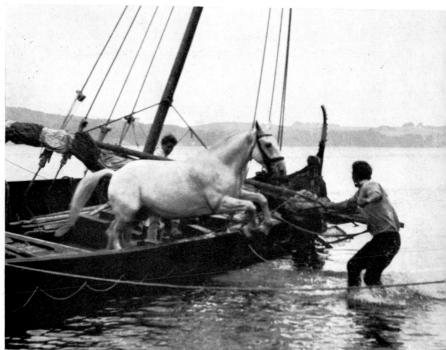

5 Detail from the Bayeux Tapestry depicting the unloading of a horse from an invasion ship. *Photo Phaidon Press.*

6 Reconstruction of the scene by Danish scouts in 1963, using a replica of the Ladby excavated in 1935 and accepted as being similar to ships used by William in 1066. *Photo Viking Ship Museum of Denmark, Roskilde.*

It has been estimated that a fleet of Viking Longships would cover an average of 40 nautical miles a day in fair summer weather. So Hardrada's travelling time between Bergen and the Orkneys would have been probably about seven days. But allowing for a lay-over in the Shetlands while slower ships caught up with the warships and the fleet re-formed, he probably reached the marvellously sheltered inner anchorages of Scapa Flow, to the north of Kirkwall, and the Westray and Stronsay Firths, on or about 14–15 September. There he picked up again some ships which had sailed directly from Norway to the Orkneys because there was no need of them in the Shetlands. They were transports and supply craft suitable for taking aboard whatever was available in the Orkneys to help fuel the long and exacting expedition to the south.

And in the Orkneys he left behind Ellisef and the two daughters. They would never see him again. But Olaf sailed south with him, along with volunteers from these lonely islands and the two earls, Paul and Erlend, sons of the great chieftain Thorfinn, who jointly ruled the Orkneys as his viceroys. Hardrada's massive sortie was now well under way. Rounding the Scottish coast off Peterhead, Aberdeen and Dundee, his fleet closed the Firth of Forth. Somewhere in these waters he made rendezvous with Tostig, who had been awaiting him with all the ships and men he had been able to muster in Flanders and Scotland to add to the remnants of his own original, mauled, raiding force. According to Hardrada's own reporters, he had left Sognes Fiord with some 200 ships, and these same sources also declare that after he had paused in the islands north of Scotland and had joined up with Tostig, his total fleet had grown into about 300 units. This estimate is confirmed in the Anglo-Saxon Chronicle and so, for once, figures given by somewhat haphazard medieval arithmeticians may reasonably be accepted. These 300 ships now sailed southwards for Northumbria, before the same northerly wind which was keeping Duke William's ships herded in St Valery. Silently, and probably too far out to sea to be observed by whatever watchers there might have been in small and lonely settlements ashore, the sinister armada stole towards its goal.

It made its first brief pause in English waters at the mouth of the Tyne. There is no word from any source that Hardrada and Tostig put men ashore here, probably because there was really nothing to plunder in this remote north-eastern outpost. The halt was probably made so that the fleet could re-form before it started

D

the serious business of the expedition; there were bound to be stragglers and minor casualties after a journey of well over 100 miles and a period of some three days and three nights spent at sea. Then southwards again headed the fleet. Two days after leaving the mouth of the Tyne Hardrada ordered the first raid upon English ground. His men surged ashore and looted and destroyed a settlement on the site of the modern region of Cleveland, in Yorkshire.

Scarborough, a day's sail further south, was the next place to suffer, and here the killings and the pillaging perpetrated by the pitiless Norwegians were greater, for Scarborough was a settlement of notable size and antiquity. It had developed on a site originally used in the late Bronze Age and subsequently enlarged by the Romans. Here was a dilapidated signal tower once used by the Romans, one of a chain built by them along the coast of Yorkshire about 370. That this particular signalling tower, meant to be fed by flares and bonfires, was usable in 1066 is unlikely, for almost everything Roman had been allowed to decay during the centuries after the invaders left England. But Scarborough had its defenders who resisted Hardrada's warriors with spirit and determination but were inevitably overwhelmed. The invaders then climbed a hill overlooking the settlement and set fire to the primitive homesteads below with long gaff-poles, after having looted them and, it seems likely, having seized some of the menfolk as slaves and conscripts, and women as concubines. It was savage treatment for a settlement which had actually been founded and named by Vikings after a raid by a force led by Thorgils Scarthi (the hare-lipped).

The Norwegian fleet next rounded Flamborough Head and slid down the flat and featureless coastline of Yorkshire like some enormous snake seeking its prey. It closed the coast several times so that the hungry invaders could replenish their stores by looting settlements in Holderness, the south-eastern plains region of the East Riding of Yorkshire. Here again from time to time they were resisted, stubbornly but hopelessly, by bands of local defenders. News of the approach of the dreaded Norwegians was at last being spread ahead of them, but if the word had reached York, the capital of the north about 50 miles inland from Flamborough Head, there had not yet been time for Earl Morcar to mobilize his fyrd and despatch it against the invaders. Nobody yet knew for certain whether Hardrada was making a limited sequence of summer raids or was intent upon fully-fledged invasion, although evidence pointing towards the greater calamity was mounting as coastal incursions were made further and further south and the enormous size of the raiding force became more widely apparent.

Hardrada and Tostig were making for the point of their permanent penetration of England – the lagoon-like mouth of the great river Humber, with its sheltered waters almost eight miles wide behind the protective, curved arm of Spurn Head. Their ultimate target was the citadel of York, the capture of which would almost certainly yield them control of the whole of north-eastern England and provide them with a great fortified base in which they could gather enough strength to meet any force which a distracted King Harold might be able to send against them. York was already a handsome city of over 1,750 houses, according to ancient records, and was second only to London in size and importance.

This was the invaders' grand strategy and as always in such military affairs there were advantages and risks in the attempt to fulfil it. Firstly, it was an advantage to them that although York was so far inland it was attainable by water, firstly via the Humber and then the Ouse. Also, it had a strong pro-Viking element in its population, for it had fallen to the invading Danes in 867 and had been given by them its permanent name, Yorvik. Further, many of the settlements in the wooded countryside between York and the sea and along the very banks of the Humber and the Ouse also had many inhabitants with Viking links and heritage. So the Norwegians could count on at least some sympathy and help as they moved inland. Tostig, for all his dubious past as earl of the region, might also be able to rally some of his fellow Anglo-Saxon northerners to the campaign of conquest. But offsetting these advantages was the handicap that now that the fleet was in the Humber it would be visible and vulnerable from both banks, increasingly so as the river narrowed and then became the much smaller Ouse halfway to York. And Morcar also had a fleet. It was tiny compared with the Norwegian one but it might be capable of stinging Hardrada's tail as he sailed westwards. And Morcar and Edwin would sooner or later mobilize to block the invader's entry into York. So far everything had gone well for Hardrada. Surprise had served him handsomely. Now that was gone, and the decisive trials of strength were at hand.

The North Resists

Whatever the warmth or otherwise of the feelings of the brother earls towards King Harold – and there seems little doubt that they cared for his preservation with about as minuscule enthusiasm as they cared for the unity of the kingdom he ruled – they resolved not to let their territories in northern and central England fall by default to Hardrada and Tostig. But because of the substantial pro-Viking affinity among their people in Northumbria and Mercia they could not have found it easy to enrol any large number of volunteers willing to fight off the invading Norwegians. However willing Edwin might have been to help his brother, who was the more urgently threatened, he was based much too far to the south to get his forces to the critical area between the mouth of the Humber and the city of York, in time to make possible an early attack upon Hardrada and Tostig which would have been strong enough to have a chance of success. Morcar's consequent numerical weakness produced an interesting sequence of naval and military tactics, really a game of manoeuvre and opportunistic evasion.

Morcar made the first move. He sent his fleet of small ships, which would have been overwhelmed in any battle in open waters with Hardrada's massive flotillas of Longships and other craft, down the Ouse to impede the passage of the invaders towards York by whatever means they could devise. The better they did this task the more time would Morcar be given to mobilize his forces, and the more time would Edwin have to do the same in Mercia and then send his troops on their ponies towards York to join Morcar in the inevitable decisive encounter with the Norwegians.

The commander of the Northumbrian ships evidently concluded that prudence was preferable to useless valour. His very presence in the Ouse ahead of Hardrada must have achieved something towards slowing down the invaders, but he seems to have made no direct assault or other challenge of any kind. He was a wise man. In the narrow waters of the Ouse he would have been in double danger since, besides opposing him in a naval fight, Hardrada would have been easily able to spare sizeable companies of his warriors to go ashore and assault the Northumbrians from the land.

The defenders fell back in their ships before the oncoming

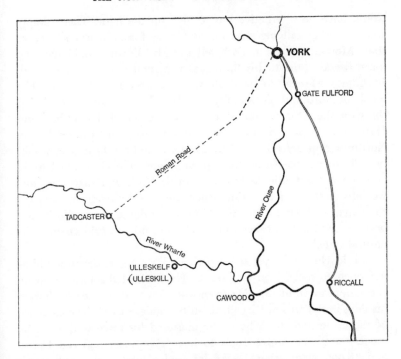

Site of the Battle of Gate Fulford. Stamford Bridge is seven miles east of York on the River Derwent.

Norwegians, who were of course masters in the practice of navigating tidal waters. But instead of taking the obvious course of continuing along the Ouse back to York the Northumbrians retreated due west long the much smaller river Wharfe, which still joins the Ouse at the village of Cawood. They sailed on in the direction of Tadcaster, already a sizeable settlement on a Roman road linking York with the midlands, and stopped short at Ulleskill, two miles to the south-east of Tadcaster. Here they moored and lay in waiting, their commander having calculated that with patience he might yet be able to use his outnumbered men and ships to advantage. He knew, of course, that Hardrada's vital objective was York, and he reasoned that Hardrada would not squander time on his way there simply to chase after a few small ships up the Wharfe. The Norwegian would be anxious to take York as quickly as he possibly could because once he occupied it the whole of the north would have no alternative but to give up the fight. There simply were no other rallying points or defensive forces of any size other than Morcar's. Also, if York fell quickly, Edwin would have no incentive to come to his brother's help, and would probably fall back into Mercia, to be dealt with at leisure on his own. The whole of Northumbria would be Hardrada's – including the lurking ships on the Wharfe. But if the assault on York languished and Hardrada's ships and men became in any way hard pressed by the Northumbrian defenders led by Morcar, then the little fleet would be able to emerge from the Wharfe, regain the Ouse at Cawood and use a flood tide to hasten towards York and take the Norwegians in the rear at a time when they were already fighting for their lives in their front. (The Ouse was tidal as far as York, and beyond, until recent times when locks and other works changed its natural state.)

Harald Hardrada was too experienced a commander to lay himself open to a fight on two fronts. He avoided the naval trap by the simple move of stepping from water on to dry land. Anchoring his ships in the area of Riccall, about two miles east of the confluence of the Ouse and the Wharfe, he mustered his force (estimated by modern military professionals to have comprised between 15,000 and 18,000 men) ashore as an impressive land army. Not all his men were fighting troops, of course. We can only make rough estimates of the proportion of non-combatants in a medieval amphibious force such as Hardrada's, but a modern consensus is that he had about 6,000 men to put into battle. Not even all these were available for the march upon York, for he had to leave some of them behind to mount guard over his ships.

He then set off with the remainder – perhaps 5,000 warriors – some proceeding along one principal track and others on a minor one passing close to the Ouse through the settlement of Stillingfleet. The total distance between Riccall and York was about ten miles, not an arduous trek for Vikings in prime physical condition. The two long columns of armed fighting men, occasionally coming within hailing distance of each other from one track to the other, trudged in the cool September air towards York, and towards the battle which they knew lay ahead of them before the citadel became theirs. One sees a few privileged men, including Hardrada and Tostig and their closest subordinates, riding on captured ponies, with the rest of the host singing, talking and bantering to keep up their spirits in the manner of soldiers throughout the ages, until the fearful technology of the twentieth century turned warfare from a dangerous adventure into a frightening ordeal for all.

Morcar followed English tradition in getting ready to meet the invaders. Unlike the people of continental states – including Normandy, where the fortified wooden castle was already a well-used stronghold – the Anglo-Saxons still preferred to fight their battles in the open field or, at best, from the top of a hill rather than from behind protective walls, or with houses and other buildings around them. All existing records show that by 1066 they had let the sturdy walls built by the Romans to enclose and seal off important places such as London, York, Chester and elsewhere, crumble away. Accordingly, Morcar did not order his Housecarls and levies to wait for the Norwegians to come upon them in the narrow, twisting alleys and small spaces between the dwellings of York. Instead, he led them, and there is no evidence on which to base an estimate of their numbers, along the main track leading to the south from the city gates and formed them into a defensive line at Gate Fulford, one mile outside York. Here the two tracks being used by the Norwegians met and became one thoroughfare running parallel to the Ouse several hundred yards east of it. Morcar dared not venture further south than Gate Fulford. To have done so would have taken him and his men beyond the junction of the two tracks and put them into the disastrous predicament of having to fight two columns of the enemy at one time.

He was able to get into his chosen battle position some hours before Hardrada and Tostig reached Gate Fulford. If this had not been so, the Norwegians would have swept through them, brushing them aside before they were established and then pushing on unopposed into York. The two armies faced each other in swampy meadows between river and road which are still identifiable close to the Ouse and between two sturdy mansions, Water Fulford Hall and Gate Fulford Hall. The site of the battle that followed is still miraculously clear of urban development, which has halted a few hundred yards north of the battleground. The area is a challenge to the civic conscience as a site for permanent preservation – an eternal reminder of an interesting fragment of Yorkshire history. Water birds wheeled and bleated in 1973 over the meadows and across the Ouse, about 80 feet wide here, and the visitor could readily conjure up the noise and turmoil of primitive battle, as he stood close to the eastern bank of the placid river and looked across the silent and empty grasslands.

Morcar had placed his men in a line several ranks deep in the usual English fashion. It ran from the easterly bank of the Ouse on his right, across the Fulford meadows in his centre and thence astride the track as far east as a ditch which was so swampy that it did not offer safe passage for a man. The way into York was blocked. Hardrada now prepared to remove this challenge to his advance by lining up his army with his best, most experienced troops on his left flank and close to him in the centre, and his weakest men on his right as far as the ditch. This was sound deployment. His left and central divisions would have the best chance of hacking a way through the English line because they were on firm ground and could not be outflanked since their extreme left was sealed off by the Ouse. He could not count upon his green troops on his right for too much. It would be satisfactory if they merely held their ground. They were facing some good soldiers – the English were acknowledged by Normans and Scandinavians alike to be among the best infantrymen in all Europe – who could not be outflanked because their left was so effectively sealed by the boggy ground. But Hardrada did have one minor asset to counter Morcar's control of the track between Fulford and his base in York. Not far behind that part of the meadowland was a ford of big stones which, local people say, was still being used until the opening of the twentieth century as a foot crossing of the Ouse. This gave Hardrada an auxiliary avenue of communication between him and his ships anchored at Riccall; and, if the day went badly, it would provide an extra escape route for his troops.

The two armies became interlocked in the customary savage physical combat of the times, with men flailing, hacking and jabbing at each other with sword, axe and spear. Snorri, the Viking chronicler, concedes that the English defenders soon gained a promising advantage. Hardrada's weakest link, the men on his right, gave way under the hefty blows of Morcar's fyrdmen, forebears of the dour and tough northcountrymen who throughout England's later history became renowned for their strength and steadfastness, as well as for the bluntness and taciturnity which accompanied these qualities. The English left began to advance dangerously along the track to the south, bending Hardrada's line back ominously. He reacted to the threat with the speed and resourcefulness for which Snorri claimed he was famous. He ordered the proven warriors on his left to spread out towards his centre while still holding firm against the English facing them. As they did so he led the men under his immediate command on a wheeling movement from the centre of his line to take the advancing English on his right in their flank. He must have enjoyed a considerable superiority in numbers over Morcar that day, for not only did his left-central divisions hold firm on an extended front but, as his chronicler reports, his own flanking charge was made by so many men that it proved 'irresistible'. The English advance stopped abruptly. The men who had been making it were split into small groups fighting side by side for their lives as they took the shock of the charge and were driven step by step eastwards towards the ditch, which had now become their enemy instead of an ally. Seeing these English giving way in increasing disorder, Hardrada's defeated troops regained their spirit and rejoined the attack against the very troops who had so recently been beating them back. Norwegian morale all along the line strengthened as the English morale sagged. Over towards the Ouse the defending line began to yield. Very soon the brief and swiftly-changing battle ended in a rout. Hardrada had won yet another victory.

The one version of the Anglo-Saxon Chronicle which gives more than passing attention to the Battle of Gate Fulford confirms the Norwegian account in outline if not in detail and concedes the total defeat of Morcar and his men. It says: 'Earl Edwin and Earl Morcar had gathered as great a force as they could from their earldom, and fought that host and made great slaughter of them; but a great number of the English were either slain or drowned or driven in flight. This battle took place on the Vigil of St Matthew the Apostle [20 September] which was a Wednesday.' Evidently some of the English managed to escape from the field. The others were driven into the Ouse or into the treacherous swamp, or were killed before they got there.

One or two points about the low-keyed and inadequate narrative in the Chronicle are worth attention. It brings Earl Edwin into the story, but the reference to him is puzzling because it implies that he was a co-earl of Northumbria with his brother Morcar, whereas he was of course Earl of Mercia, with vast territories to the south of Northumbria. Slipping in the name of Edwin may have represented a rather muddled attempt to enlarge the role played by the

House of Leofric, to which Edwin and Morcar belonged, in trying to resist the invader. The edition of the Chronicle concerned is the one which is consistently partisan to that House and antagonistic to the rival House of Godwin. Other editions of the Chronicle which were simply copied from this version also state of course that Earl Edwin was at Fulford but their evidence is worthless. Perhaps Edwin saw the emergency which threatened his brother and also realized that he could not raise a significant army of his own in time to help Morcar; so he and whatever bodyguard and Housecarls were available raced north to York and were in time to join the battle.

Whatever the truth, the defeat obliterated the brothers as factors in the whirl of events during the rest of the year. They simply disappeared temporarily from the national stage. Indeed, their record for the rest of their lives is one of weakness and indecision. It would seem certain that neither was of a calibre appropriate to his high rank – one the lord of one-quarter of England in the north and the other of the central area stretching from one coast to the other and embracing most of the southern and north-western midlands. The military performance at Gate Fulford was typically undistinguished, to rate it at its highest. The only excusing circumstance was that Morcar's forces were outnumbered but even this may be interpreted as a reproach, for Morcar should surely have been able to muster an army big enough to have halted an invading force which had had to cross many hundreds of miles by water and had no established base in the alien country it was despoiling. One can still criticize Morcar on this score despite the existence of a pro-Viking faction within his earldom, for he had been determinedly sought and accepted by the people of the north only a year earlier as successor to the hated Tostig, who was now trying to re-impose himself upon them under the patronage of Harald Hardrada.

Victory at Fulford yielded York to Hardrada and Tostig. It also gave them a heady indication that their scheme for the conquest and division of England might not be very difficult to fulfil, for the resistance to them so far had been pitifully inadequate. They must have been in high spirits between the Wednesday and the Sunday of that third week in September. The civic administrators of the city of York hastened to make terms with Hardrada, and abject terms they were. He was to be granted undisputed control of the city, to take from it whatever he needed, and its leaders and population were to recognize him as their king and help him to oust

Harold from the rest of the kingdom. As the Chronicle records, 'Harald and Tostig agreed to conclude an abiding peace with the citizens provided that they all marched southwards with him to conquer the realm.' In return for the prompt and complete capitulation and the wholesale promise of help to come, Hardrada agreed not to damage York or loot it of any of its treasures as was the usual Viking custom, but in refraining from doing so he was actually serving himself. He could see that he would probably need York as a base and a shelter for his army and his ships, not only during the coming operations in the north but probably for at least part of the winter. He knew from King Harold's record and reputation as a soldier that here was no feeble Morcar but a resolute and skilled campaigner, and once he had been dealt with, there would probably be another challenger to meet – Duke William of Normandy. Hardrada needed all the English help he could get.

At this stage everything was still going splendidly for him. While he and Tostig went through the formalities of negotiations with the administrators of York, his victorious but weary troops could go back to the ships at Riccall for some rest and recreation, for there appeared to be no immediate threat, from King Harold or anybody else, of interference with the enjoyment of the rewards of victory at Gate Fulford. Hardrada and Tostig therefore spent two, perhaps three days arranging to take over York and then followed their troops back to Riccall, having settled upon Monday, 25 September, as the date for the return of hostages mutually given and the settlement of the final details of the permanent armistice. Stamford Bridge, eight miles east-north-east of York, was decided upon as the most convenient place for the culminating conference. The choice of Stamford Bridge, which had developed on or close to the site of a Roman encampment called Delgovitia, was good for several reasons. It was well distant from the city of York, where the proposed meeting would have encumbered streets and buildings and, if it went wrong, might very well have been followed by a bloody massacre of the inhabitants by Hardrada's bodyguards and troops. Stamford Bridge was also much closer to Riccall than York and was consequently much more convenient to the victors. Further, it was an important communications centre, having roads or tracks leading to it from all four principal points of the compass, including a good track which Hardrada and Tostig and their men could use for the pony ride or walk of about 12 miles from the ships at

Riccall. The other roads would make it easy for landowners, thegns and other notables living in the Yorkshire Wolds, the Vale of Pickering and the spreading valley east of York to attend the Monday meeting and, as Hardrada could confidently expect, enrol on the side of the winner. These areas were, according to the Domesday survey, among the most thickly populated in the whole of northern England in 1066; their enlistment into the territory of the invaders would be one of the valuable fruits of the victory at Gate Fulford. Hardrada and Tostig could justifiably look forward to an enjoyable day at Stamford Bridge, on Monday, 25 September.

6

Harold's Finest Victory

The affairs of men are rarely so dazzlingly prosperous as they seem, and rarely so bleak : sometimes when they seem at their peak, and securely so, they are actually about to plunge to the bottom. So it was to be with Harald Hardrada, the ever-victorious warrior, and Tostig, the tormented outcast. During the four days after their stirring triumph at Gate Fulford they were at the very height of their careers. On the fifth day they went to their eternal doom.

King Harold, their Nemesis, is assumed to have had his fears confirmed that the Norwegian assault upon England was an invasion and not simply another temporary Viking incursion, within a week of the burning of Scarborough. That ghastly event, which occurred some time during the first two weeks of September, told Harold the real story. The raids on Cleveland and Holderness had been small and, it could reasonably be supposed, merely pinpricks at a moment when England was divided and distraught, her new King weak and threatened. But after Scarborough there was no doubt what was afoot. After firing that settlement the Viking ships had once again turned south instead of loading their plunder and heading back towards the Orkneys and home. They must now be treated as containing a threat to the kingdom itself.

The only means for this disturbing news to be carried to Harold was by human messenger. Men would have to ride well over 200 miles through the heart of the country to reach Harold at London, Winchester, or wherever he was waiting and watching for Duke William's coming. They would make the journey on ponies and the shortest possible time would be four days, perhaps five. We can imagine these bodes pressing on south, perhaps making the long journey in relays to save time, along the tracks and overgrown Roman roads running through the densely wooded and sparsely peopled shires of the midlands and the south – almost unbelievably different from today's teeming industrial hives, cleared fields and downlands and wide motorways filled with too many vehicles. Not all the changes during nine centuries have been for the better, and we should pause before condemning the men of 1066 for their savagery and pitying them for their ignorance and primitiveness.

Harold now faced a choice which could very well determine the future of his kingdom. He could stay where he was, in the south, to go on waiting for William until all possibility of a Channel crossing and a landing had gone until next year. If he made this choice he would be hoping that Edwin and Morcar were capable at least of holding Hardrada and Tostig in check, even if they could not destroy the invaders, until Duke William had been dealt with by Harold or had failed to appear. Then Harold could go north at a time and pace of his own choice with an army big enough to be certain of crushing the Norwegians. The alternative was to gamble that Duke William would not invade for another month. Harold could then hasten north to Yorkshire with his Housecarls and whatever volunteers and conscripts he could gather about him and, taking Hardrada by surprise, achieve an immediate victory over him. Then he could safely turn about and hurry back to his southern bases in case William should still find it possible to cross the Channel before the winter closed in. Everything we know about Harold indicates that the second choice would be the one to appeal to him. He was sanguine and impetuous, not a man to sit back and wait.

How much he knew at this time of William's situation and intentions on the other side of the Channel is debatable. It is to be suspected, however, that either he knew very little or had been fed false information through the Norman and pro-Norman local magnates living in south-east England. Otherwise, even allowing for his temperament, he would not have elected to dash northwards at the very moment when William was poised to sail for Sussex from St Valery as soon as the long-overdue change of wind came and gave him his opportunity. Yet he did so and, in the short term, everything went far more favourably for him than he could have hoped. Only in the long term did he have to pay full forfeit for his brilliant impetuosity.

Having made his decision he wasted no time in putting it into effect. After nine months of uncertainty, frustration and inactivity, he and his Housecarls, men who were trained to fight and had little other purpose in life except to do so, must have been longing to move somewhere, against somebody. King and army set out for Yorkshire on their ponies on 20 September. It was the very day on which Morcar's army was being routed at Gate Fulford, but Harold knew nothing of any such encounter, of course. He could have known very little about what had happened since Hardrada and Tostig led their ships into the Humber, and this lack of news may have been one of the factors which helped him to decide to go north. But he needed no confirmation that York was their eventual target.

Riding hard, picking up stores and maybe some volunteers as he went, Harold achieved one of the outstanding feats of military manoeuvrability in medieval times in taking an army of at least 6,000 armed warriors on a ride of about 200 miles through central England in four days. To cover an average of about 50 miles a day with such a mass of men was a truly phenomenal performance. He had the advantage of not being encumbered with a large number of non-combatants and slow supply elements, for he was traversing country over which he had supreme authority, even if he did not command the unanimous friendliness of its inhabitants, and he could ride confidently forward with his Housecarls, knowing that he could commandeer whatever they needed as they rode on and also knowing that the slower people following them would certainly be able to catch up with them within 24 hours after the journey to York was done. Harold's army clattered into Tadcaster, ten miles south of York and so within easy reach of it, on Sunday, 24 September. Here again was an Anglo-Saxon community established on the site of a Roman settlement (known then as Calcaria). Tadcaster had grown around a point where the Roman road or track which Harold had been following through the West Riding of Yorkshire reached the southerly bank of the river Wharfe, only two miles from where Morcar's lurking small fleet was still moored. Here was an excellent spot for Harold's weary men to rest and refurbish while he gathered all possible information on which to determine his next move. Here were lush, low-lying meadows where men and horses could lie at ease sheltered from the winds of early autumn. Today one can still find such a meadow just below the ancient parish church of St Mary – grassland sloping down to the Wharfe, fresh water in abundance tumbling over the small rocks, even a ford of stepping stones across the river. This is a spot almost

surely used by Harold's warriors when they came into Tadcaster that
September day in 1066.

Tadcaster was also a place where Harold could quickly catch
up on all that had happened while he had been riding so hard
from the distant south. Everybody would know the grim news of the
defeat of Morcar's army. The sailors at Ulleskill could tell him that
Hardrada and Tostig had now gone back to their ships at Riccall
after their entry into York. Travellers who had been in York knew
of the capitulation and the negotiations that had followed it and
had not yet ended. He learned, and this was the most important
news, of the final parley to be held next day at Stamford Bridge.
Now he could easily assess the situation and the possibilities it
offered him, in spite of its depressing nature. Once again he was
faced with alternatives. He could stay overnight in Tadcaster and
muster his rested men before dawn for a ride or march of some ten
miles to Riccall, to pounce upon the unsuspecting Norwegians while
they were still abed. As likely as not they would be besotted with the
aftermath of their victory parties and drinking, and with luck his
Housecarls would be able to make short work of them before they
knew what had overwhelmed them. Or, he could wait a little
longer the next morning and attack the Norwegians from the flank
while they were walking and riding to the rendezvous at Stamford
Bridge. Or, he could go into York next morning to re-assert the
English royal authority and order the local administrators to stay
at home while he and his army went in their stead to meet
Hardrada and Tostig at Stamford Bridge.

This last alternative clearly offered Harold the best chance of
carrying out his aim of crushing the invasion quickly and thoroughly
and it was the one that he decided to use. The two others had flaws
and risks which reduced their appeal. An attack upon the base
at Riccall might not secure the hoped-for complete surprise because
the Norwegians, however confident and at ease they might be,
could very well have posted sentries around their ships and encampments and some of these might have just enough time before
the slaughter developed to give an alarm. The flank attack on the
way to Stamford Bridge was more attractive, but it also had some
drawbacks. One of these was that since the Norwegians would be on
their way to a peaceful parley, with no thought of battle in their
minds, they would probably straggle in small parties towards the
rendezvous and would consequently be hard to attack effectively;

in these circumstances Harold's Housecarls would probably also
not be able to attack without giving away their presence very
early and provoke a quick general alarm which would frustrate the
concept of surprise inherent in the manoeuvre. The third alternative plan of pouncing upon the Norwegians at Stamford Bridge
seemed to have none of these handicaps. The sudden attack would
find the Norwegians isolated from their base, unorganized and at
ease, without their full equipment of weapons close at hand, and
lulled into sluggishness because they were expecting harmless civilian
negotiators instead of an avenging host such as Harold's.

One precaution Harold had to take that Sunday in Tadcaster
and, according to the Norwegian scribes who gave the most detailed
account of what happened, he did not neglect it. This was to make
sure that not a hint about his unexpected arrival there seeped out
to Hardrada and Tostig at Riccall. He achieved this by posting
guards at all the exits and entrances of the town and at strategic
points along the highways leading out of it towards York and
alongside the Ouse towards Ulleskill and Riccall. He appears to
have been completely successful in sealing off Tadcaster. What is
not clear is the timing of his move from Tadcaster to York. The
one edition of the Anglo-Saxon Chronicle which mentions it says
without qualification : 'And on the Monday he marched into York.'
But Snorri reports with equal certainty that he rode into York on
the Sunday night and adds : 'This army was in the town during the
night.' There is no way of settling this contradiction, but what is
not disputed is that Harold was certainly in York very early on the
Monday morning. He needed time for negotiation in the city before
going on to Stamford Bridge. He does not seem to have had too
much difficulty in the city, for there is no mention anywhere of
any military or other resistance to him. We might assume that his
highly dramatic and unexpected arrival at the head of a formidable
force, plus the effect of the physical presence in the north of an
English king (a rare event indeed in this region) and perhaps also
the sway exercized by his own strong personality won the administrators away from their shameful surrender to Hardrada and caused
them to decide promptly and unequivocally for Harold, in spite of
the oath they had given so recently to Hardrada.

The day was still not far advanced when Harold and his thousands of Housecarls and other troops set out along a Roman road out
of York on the short journey of eight miles east-north-east to

Stamford Bridge; for seven of those miles they followed the same course as do modern travellers. Harold knew the time of the planned meeting, of course, and it would seem that he got his men to Gate Helmsley, a halt on the Roman road just over a mile from Stamford Bridge but not visible from there, shortly before the relaxed invaders began to assemble casually on both sides of the bridge over the river Derwent. Then he gave the word to advance. Housecarls and militiamen began to move down the slight hill from Gate Helmsley to Stamford Bridge. The September sun was casting its golden rays upon them and, as Snorri records, 'the shining arms of the English were like glinting ice to the eyes' of the astonished Norwegians. The surprise achieved by Harold was total. It is an impressive disclosure of the difference between the world of today and that of 1066 that Harold had only to use the simplest precautions to shift his warriors over an area now occupied by many tens of thousands of people without his enemy even having learned that he had left the south, much less that he was only a mile away and advancing to the attack.

Hardrada and Tostig had only a few minutes in which to sound an alarm and array their men into some kind of battle order before Harold and his army were upon them. Hardrada could never before in his career as a soldier have been caught so unprepared and in so vulnerable a situation. He had even allowed many of his men to leave behind at Riccall their birnies (long leather coats studded with round metal bosses worn in battle by both Vikings and English) because the day was so hot, and they were going, after all, merely for a day out to a parley with unarmed civilians who had already undertaken to submit to them. 'They were very merry,' says Snorri, revealingly. Worse still, Hardrada had also left behind at Riccall about one-third of his total force to guard his fleet against guerillas and a possible raid by the Northumbrian ships still stationed a few miles away at Ulleskill. Among those who had the good fortune to have been left at Riccall that day were the two young earls of Orkney and Hardrada's young son Olaf. The man who had been left in charge of the base was Eystein Orre, a brother of Hardrada's concubine, Thora, to whom he had promised in marriage Maria, his daughter by his legal wife Ellisef. This betrothal sounds incestuous but of course it is not so. It is rather another indication of the scarcity of suitable spouses for members of the royal and noble families of the day, who were intent upon keeping relationships – and power – within as closely-linked a network of people as possible. Almost everybody within that network was related in some degree to everybody else.

Not having thought even for a moment of the possibility of combat at Stamford Bridge, Hardrada had no plan for coping with it. There is no record to suggest that he had ever before been to Stamford Bridge and he had almost certainly not surveyed the neighbouring terrain for its military possibilities and pitfalls. Tostig, who knew not only the area but also Harold's skill as a commander and the fighting qualities of his men, urged Hardrada not to give battle. Men who were with the pair that day and survived to tell the tale reported later that during the brief period while the English were coming forward from Gate Helmsley Tostig suggested urgently to Hardrada that they wheel about and retreat as fast as they could to Riccall so that they could rally there and, strengthened by the force already at the base, meet Harold on far more even terms. The suggestion sounded plausible, but Hardrada immediately turned it down. He had at least two very good reasons for doing so. The Norwegians could not hope to be able to reach Riccall without being attacked on their flanks and rear by Harold's pursuing Housecarls, who would certainly force battle upon them. Also, Harold would surely send some of his men ahead across country to seize a crossing of the Derwent, at Kexby, which the Norwegians would have to use on their way back to Riccall. And of course, retreat in any form was not at all to the liking of a man such as Harald Hardrada.

Instead of accepting what he considered to be Tostig's rather panicky suggestion, he decided to stay and fight but at the same time he sent messengers hastening back to Eystein Orre to tell him what was happening and ordering him to come to Stamford Bridge as fast as he could with all the fighting men available at the base. Then he turned to meet with his characteristic resilience and resourcefulness the extreme emergency which had come upon him. Leaving one detachment of his men to fight as a rearguard on the northern side of the Derwent and to block the passage of Harold's Housecarls across the narrow wooden bridge spanning the river, which was about 60 feet wide at this point, Hardrada led the rest of his men to the most favourable defensive ground which offered close at hand. This was a gently rising meadow which has since yielded bones, skeletons and rusted weapons to confirm the name of Battle Flats which it has borne for centuries and still does today. On a ridge dominating the meadow about 300 yards south-east of the Derwent Hardrada lined up a shield-wall of his best-armed troops during the precious time gained for him while his rearguard were disputing the crossing of the bridge.

As so often happens when the course of a confused and spread-out battle is recalled later, one incident in the first moments of the battle of Stamford Bridge was built up by survivors and has found its way into the history books. About a century after the battle, somebody who had been told the story added it to the annal for 1066 in the Abingdon edition of the Anglo-Saxon Chronicle. It appears nowhere else in contemporary primary narratives, but there seems no reason to disbelieve that something of the kind did happen. The entry in the Chronicle reads: 'But there was one Norwegian who stood firm against the English forces, so that they could not cross the bridge, nor clinch victory. An Englishman shot with an arrow but to no avail, and another went under the bridge and stabbed him through under the coat of mail. Then Harold, King of the English, crossed the bridge and his levies went forward with him.' Such are the bare outlines of the story. It is not known who added it to the Chronicle, but the man was probably not a learned scribe or even a monk, for the spelling and style are inferior to the rest of the entries in the Chronicle. The entry is not written in the usual old English but in a curious mixture of English and Latin. The story was embellished as the centuries passed, until we can find ourselves reading today that this prodigious Norwegian killed more than 40 of the English with his Viking axe and that showers of arrows did not fell him. Then, relate some modern storytellers, one Englishman put out into the river in a small boat, or maybe a salting tub, and with a swift jab of his spear upwards through a space in the boards of the bridge brought the heroic defender to excruciating and humiliating death. Yet another embellishment, added several centuries after the grisly event, was that King Harold, seeing the inspiring prowess of the lone Norwegian on the bridge, halted the attack upon him to offer him honourable passage through the English lines if he would give up his hopeless defence and let the attackers through. Of course, the Norwegian scorned the offer and killed still more Englishmen before the dastardly blow dispatched him. It could have happened so, but obviously did not.

Snorri also beclouds the facts about Stamford Bridge with another tale which cannot be dismissed outright as fantasy because it too *could* have happened, although commonsense suggests strongly that it did not, at least in the romantic form produced by the fluent bard. He says that before the battle proper began, presumably after the tussle for the bridge had ended, a small party of envoys rode out under a truce flag from the assembling English ranks, sought out Tostig and offered terms under which the coming clash could be averted. Their spokesman said that King Harold would give back the earldom of Northumbria to Tostig if he would forsake Hardrada, the foreign invader, and return to the English fold. A further possibility was that Harold might even offer Tostig dominion in one-third of all England if the restoration of his earldom did not suit him or was not enough for him.

'And what will he give Harald Hardrada?' Tostig is said to have asked. 'Seven feet of English ground, or a little more since he is taller than other men,' the envoy answered. Snorri says the bargain was spurned by Tostig because he would not think of deserting his ally. Only after the envoys had gone back into the English lines did Tostig tell Hardrada, according to Snorri, that the man who had offered the terms had been King Harold himself. Hardrada thereupon declared it was a pity that he had not known this because if he had, he would have made sure that the King did not get away from him; and he added musingly : 'He is a small man but he sits firmly in his saddle.' Such is Snorri's story and it reads very like one of those pieces of verbal romancing of which he was fond. Possibly the basis for it was that some approach was made to Tostig by Harold that day in the hope of isolating Hardrada, but it would hardly have been made by the king in person or in the form related. Harold would be most unlikely to risk placing himself physically at the mercy of the brother who had shown such hatred of him and had already done him so much harm since January. Nor would he jeopardize his position as king and his brand new association with the people of York by undertaking to impose Tostig for a second time upon subjects who had so recently thrown him out. Finally, the whole purpose of his embassy at Stamford Bridge – to settle everything without bloodshed – would surely have been frustrated by the cynical and harsh insult flung at Harald Hardrada; it would have stung him into fighting all the more fiercely even if Tostig had given in to the temptation to desert him.

Snorri's fancy tale is in keeping with his lamentable performance as a historian in describing the battle of Stamford Bridge as a whole. His narrative betrays his reliance on old soldiers' notoriously distorted and exaggerated accounts of what happened, his ignorance of the geography of the region, and above all the surprising confusion in his mind as to which battle in England he was describing. He was also naturally biassed in favour of Hardrada and Tostig, although to do him justice he did try to offset this with references to English bravery. His motive in dramatizing, or even inventing, the story of Harold's offer to Tostig may well have been to counter the blackness of the reputation held by Tostig in England and Normandy. This is strongly suggested by the statement he puts into Tostig's mouth that he was no murderer and that if there were to be any treachery that day he would rather be the loser than the gainer – a most unlikely declaration by the Tostig we know. But Tostig was of Viking stock and a friend and ally of the great Harald Hardrada. He would be suitably fulfilling both roles, in Snorri's mind, by stoutly refusing to desert Hardrada in a moment of supreme need.

As with so many events in medieval history, it is a pity that Snorri, or preferably somebody else with a more practical and precise mind, did not go to York and Stamford Bridge to talk with people who knew or took part in what went on in 1066. But nobody did so, and the best we can do now is to roam the area and build up, on the undisputed facts, a credible picture of what happened. Taking into consideration discoveries which have been made in succeeding centuries, we can make sober deductions on what the late Lieutenant-Colonel Alfred Burne described so graphically as 'inherent military probability'. The first and possibly most important impression which such a study produces is that the battle was a much bigger affair than is indicated by the cursory attention it has been given by historians, chiefly because it was almost immediately dwarfed by the infinitely more decisive Battle of Hastings. The number of troops involved, certainly on the English side, was in all probability higher than at Hastings. The fighting was bitter and prolonged and casualties appear to have been extraordinarily high judging by the number of leading figures who fell. The Housecarls who also fell that day could not possibly have been replaced within three weeks for use by Harold at Hastings. Secondly, Harald Hardrada was greatly outnumbered, possibly by a margin of two to one, and it is a melancholy tribute to the wild valour of the Norwegians that for at least four hours they fought savagely until they dropped, as the greater number of Englishmen pitted against them took the inevitable toll. Thirdly, this overwhelming but weakening victory which appeared to justify King Harold's head-strong dash into the northcountry was in fact as powerful a factor as any other in ensuring his defeat at Hastings so soon afterwards. Fourthly, it was the last battle fought in England in which cavalry was not used.

The first phase of the battle ended when the English swarmed over the bridge on the heels of the retreating invaders. Once over it – and to this day historians are still debating whether or no it stood where the present bridge stands or some 250 yards upstream – Harold's warriors formed themselves into a long line several ranks deep at the foot of the meadow sloping up from the south bank of the Derwent. There they regrouped, filling the gaps left by their dead and wounded, and prepared for the next stage – an assault upon the surviving Norwegians, who by this time were similarly deployed along the ridge at the top of Battle Flats. When his attacking force was ready, the freshest troops in the front line and reserves banked up behind them, Harold gave the order to advance up the slope. There would be trumpets and shouting and then the familiar awesome clash and clatter of two seemingly irresistible walls of armed men meeting head-on. The fighters hacking and slashing at each other this September afternoon could not know it, but this was to be the last time that the traditional infantryman battle would be fought in England; and it was also the last time that Viking raiders tried to assert their power over any part of England.

The battle went much more badly for the Norwegians than Hardrada could have expected, but he never knew just how badly, for he was struck down, fatally wounded, apparently very early in the combat, in circumstances which are still unclear. Snorri continues his poor performance as a war reporter by recording that Hardrada fell with an arrow in the throat. This is unlikely since the English rarely used archers except to cover an advance towards the enemy's wall of shields, and the suspicion must be entertained that Snorri, who was writing many years after 1066, had heard about the Battle of Hastings and had picked up some garbled version of the story that King Harold had been felled there by an arrow in the eye, and had once again confused the battles and the victims. It is more likely that Hardrada was killed by an English axe or javelin. However he died, his collapse from his traditional position close to his battle standard in the thick of the fight must have shaken the spirits of the Norwegians fighting against odds along the ridge, but there is no evidence whatever that they wavered. Nor did they appear to weaken when at some later stage Tostig, who had taken command after Hardrada's death, was himself struck down.

The fact that the two leaders of the defending force were killed apparently soon after one another is a token of the ferocity of the battle and the inroads which the English were making into the Norwegian line. Commanders of armies were always well covered by members of their household corps and it may be taken as certain that many of these elite soldiers were slaughtered with their captains. These bodyguards were held in special esteem in Scandinavia and in England and Normandy. They acquired social and political prestige as well as indirect power in much the same manner as do dignitaries and officials close to a monarch – the 'friends at court' of people seeking favours or concessions. It is not surprising therefore, that Snorri should make a point of naming the soldier who stood closest to Harald Hardrada at Stamford Bridge. In describing how Hardrada marshalled his force on the ridge, Snorri wrote: 'King Harald then ordered his banner, Land Ravager, to be set up, and Fredrik was the name of him who bore the banner.' He does not go on to record Fredrik's fate, but it may be imagined.

There were several good reasons why the commander of an army should be closely guarded and preserved even at the cost of many lives among his guards. The most important was not the obvious one that he directed tactics and gave all the pivotal orders, for these functions could readily be taken over by his deputy, but that his death spread dismay throughout his army in the field and gave a corresponding uplift to the enemy. So the double success of the English in despatching both Hardrada and Tostig meant that the end of the battle was inevitable, unless the Norwegians either had some unexpected compensating success or were reinforced while there was still fight left in them. The death of Tostig confirmed that the English by this time were pressing so closely that the defending shield wall was breaking up. Usually in such circumstances a battle quickly degenerated into a rout. But these stubborn Vikings – far from home and with everything to gain if they could grab a last-minute victory – did not turn and flee even though they were left virtually leaderless. They seem to have been still resisting Harold's tiring warriors in small groups by the time Eystein Orre and his reinforcements at last reached the battlefield. These men had made a forced march and ride from Riccall, however, and they were too spent and perhaps also too few to stay the triumphant English. They tried to make a fight of it, for Eystein Orre was among those killed late in the day, to no avail. The battle ended with straggling Norwegian survivors making their way back to the ships at Riccall as best they could with the English on their heels.

The scope of King Harold's victory at Stamford Bridge, his greatest and his last, is emphasized by the story of the chroniclers that when all the wounded and the stragglers surviving from the battle and pursuit were eventually rounded up they filled only 24 of the ships in which Hardrada and Tostig had brought their invasion force into England in such high hope less than a month ago. Harold treated the vanquished remnant with compassion. He gave quarter to all. They included Olaf, the non-combatant young son of Hardrada, a bishop who had been the spiritual minister to the invaders, the two younger co-earls of Orkney who had taken no part in the fighting, and the sailors who had been lucky enough to have been left behind at Riccall and had survived the last hot-blooded assault of the English upon the naval base.

Harold's men had seized the fleet after subduing some final gasps of resistance apparently burning some of the ships whose crews showed fight, and had captured all the surviving Norwegians. At a final parley held ashore at Riccall Harold demanded an oath from Olaf on behalf of all the prisoners that never again would they take up arms against England or otherwise support an expedition upon her territory. After obtaining this assurance, Harold let them go. The bodies of Hardrada and others, but not Tostig's, were put aboard the ships and eventually the pitiful collection of 24 vessels formed up for the voyage to the Orkneys and home, at a place which was then known as Ravenser. It has been identified as Ravenspur, which stood at the southernmost tip of Spurn Head, on the mouth of the Humber, but has been overrun by the encroaching North Sea at some period during succeeding centuries.

Norman scribes writing over 50 years after the Battle of Stamford Bridge pursued their post mortem vilification of Harold by asserting that he became so vain and selfish after his great triumph that he did not follow custom by dividing the spoils of battle with the troops who had fought so hard and handsomely for him. John Milton, prosecuting his own evangelical crusade that the English lost their kingdom to Duke William in 1066 because of their ungodliness, adopted and enlarged the Norman story by writing in 1640: 'Wherewith Harold, lifted up in minde, and forgetting now his former shews of popularitie, defrauded his soldiers their due and well-deserved share of the spoils.'

It all sounds malicious and untrue, out of keeping with Harold's character. He had many faults, but fairness and generosity seem to have been among his qualities judging by most of the known facts of his record. His treatment of Olaf and the defeated Norwegians belies the tale of his reputed selfishness – and short-sightedness – towards his warriors, including his own Housecarls. To treat them badly was something which an experienced commander would not do, especially one in Harold's position of knowing that his survival as king depended heavily upon the loyalty and goodwill of his soldiers. He also knew that before very long he would have to ask them for an even greater effort than they had made at Stamford Bridge because of the sure threat presented by William of Normandy. A satisfactory explanation for his withholding of plunder, which consisted largely of the stores aboard the Norwegian ships and of course the ships themselves, may be given. It is that Harold was faced not only with the certainty of an invasion later in the year or in the spring of 1067 but also with the unpleasant handicap arising from the enforced dispersal of his own fleet on 8 September and the loss of many ships in a gale while they were struggling towards the mouth of the Thames from the south coast. So he shrewdly decided to keep the Norwegian ships at readiness in the hope that he would be given enough time to muster crews to take them down to London and thence to whatever parts of the coasts of Kent and Sussex would place them to best advantage for use against William.

Let us put ourselves for a moment in Harold's position. October was at hand and the invasion season was ending. He could reasonably calculate that if William did not cross the Channel within, say, two weeks he would not invade at all this year. Accordingly Harold could argue that he would need the Norwegian ships and their stores, equipment and crews only for those two weeks; he would have plenty of time during the winter to reorganize all his defences against an invasion in the spring. So he probably did not defraud his soldiers but told them to be patient until the Norman invasion had either been postponed or had been met and overcome, and then claim and receive their rewards. After all (he could point out to them), if William landed in England and were not beaten back there would be nothing for any Englishman who still lived.

Harold led his victorious men back to York while a start was made at Riccall on preparing the Norwegian ships as quickly as possible for their journey down the east coast. We can imagine some of the thoughts and feelings which coursed in his mind as he did so. There was sadness, offset and probably outweighed by stern realism, at the death of his brother and his own share of responsibility in it. Tostig's body went to York to be buried there; no record states whether Harold was in attendance. Compensating for this perhaps unwilling sadness was his pride and thankfulness that his coup in taking Hardrada so devastatingly by surprise had obliterated one threat to his kingdom. But his defensive sword had been blunted by the loss of so many of his fine Housecarls and his obvious inability to replace them before winter. And he must have felt many pangs of disquiet at finding himself still in York, 190 miles from London and over 250 miles from the south coast, while William still had time to land.

York and the rest of the north would doubtless submit without reservation to Harold now that he had made himself the unchallenged master of the region, but it would probably not be able to offer him much in the way of military help to replace his recent losses. Hardrada and Tostig had clearly taken all the fight out of Morcar and Edwin by the debacle at Gate Fulford. What of the rest of England now? He could still count on the loyalty and support of the people in his own great former earldom of Wessex, lying between Kent and Cornwall, and upon help from the neighbouring smaller earldoms of his brothers Leofwin, Gyrth and Waltheof. But Wales was still downright hostile and would be unmoved by his victory over the Norwegians, Mercians would not desert their Earl Edwin in any great numbers, and Malcolm of Scotland would not have given up plotting and hoping to grab the furthest northern territory of England if adversity struck Harold in the south. Taking everything into account, the king's only certain salvation would come if William failed to invade this autumn. This would give him a respite of at least six months in which to strengthen his hold upon England and the English and place himself once for all in a secure military position by land and water so that he could face with confidence whatever assault might occur. Time – that, above all – was what Harold needed. It was not to be granted him.

The English scribes relate that York accepted him promptly, as he had expected now that he was a victor, and that its leaders joined him in newfound amity during the last two or three days of September. Some of the chroniclers say that he was at a feast celebrating his victory at Stamford Bridge when the news he least wished to hear came to him – that William had landed near Hastings. He had done so on the morning of 28 September, only three days after Harold's hard-fought elimination of Hardrada and Tostig.

He had the news by 1 October at the latest. No general of his experience and quality, and one in a permanent invasion-alert, could possibly have come north without having arranged some form of quick communication. This was probably something such as a chain of beacons or similar forms of signal in place of the usual mounted bodes, or perhaps even a combination of signal and human messenger to bridge areas where woodlands and hills blocked the reading of beacons, and would ensure that he heard within minimum time about any incursion in the south. We do not know how he received the news, but within hours he and all his able-bodied troops were on their way towards London, on another of those brilliant forced rides which were his and their speciality.

7

The Duke Invades

It is tempting to assume that William set sail with his fleet from St Valery during the afternoon of 27 September because he knew that two days earlier Harold had been gravely weakened by the annihilating victory he had gained over Hardrada and Tostig, and that he was geographically off balance so far to the north of England. The temptation is the greater because of the proven cleverness of William as tactician and military leader. But it is none the less a false assumption.

We could produce with confidence an array of facts which William did know on 27 September about the situation in England, but knowledge of the Battle of Stamford Bridge could not be among them. In the eleventh century, and for quite a while afterwards, there were no means whereby news could travel from York to London and thence to the south coast and across the English Channel to St Valery in two days. William could not possibly have heard the news from Stamford Bridge in 48 hours. As Professor Brooks points out in his booklet on the battle, it took some 36 hours for news of Guy Fawkes's Gunpowder Plot for blowing up the Houses of Parliament to travel from London to York in 1605, five and a half centuries later.

William did know, of course, that Harold had had to disband his militia and withdraw his fleet to London, with serious loss of ships, after 8 September. He could therefore assume that the Channel stretching out in front of him from St Valery was probably empty and that the coast, invisible to him beyond the autumn mists, was at best only lightly defended. He also knew that Hardrada had invaded and that Harold and his army had surged north to confront him, for the news of the invasion which had reached Harold from Yorkshire on or about 18 September would certainly have been relayed to William within nine days, by his own spies and resident agents in London and southern England, if by no one else. One further item of news which might also have reached him by 27 September was the encounter between the Scandinavian invaders and the forces of Morcar at Gate Fulford on 20 September. There could have been just time enough for that.

Even though ignorant of the further impressive advantage which Stamford Bridge had given him in diverting and weakening Harold, William knew enough to tell him that the period between 8 September and the end of October at the latest offered him a heaven-sent opportunity to gain a foothold in southern England, with virtual certainty of doing so at minimum and possibly negligible cost. Harold would be in no condition to make any immediate challenge. But William could perceive as clearly as could Harold that if he were given a winter of respite the King might well be able to strengthen his hold upon the country to such effect that he would be a dangerous and possibly invulnerable antagonist by the spring. His hasty gamble in riding north to wipe out the Norwegian invasion would thereby be justified, for the chances were that after the disaster at Stamford Bridge no Viking chief would make a move against England for a very long time, possibly for ever, and Harold would have only one enemy – William himself – to meet. For William it was a case of now or never. Everything had been moving in his favour since the spring of 1066, as if some beneficent god of luck had been working only for him and always against Harold. How long would the phenomenal sequence last? Calculating and suspicious, William knew better than most men of his time the fickleness of fate.

His realization of his advantages is confirmed by evidence of his eagerness to move out from St Valery, and his frustration at not being able to do so because of the contrary winds and weather. The evidence comes from the surviving reports of his own chroniclers, notably from that most privileged of the contemporary scribes, William of Poitiers. 'He made pious and fervent supplication that the wind which was still adverse might be made favourable to him, and to this end he caused the body of St Valery himself, that beloved confessor of God, to be brought outside the church,' wrote the soldier-priest. 'And all those aspiring to set out on the invasion joined with him in this act of Christian humility.' The scribe neglects to describe the exact nature of the ceremonial outside the church. But William was a pious man and his crusade had been approved and blessed by the Pope; it is likely that he made an impressive appeal to Heaven. One sees him as a man who would regard it as only right and proper that God should and would confirm the Pope.

Militarily, his need was a very specific one. Pevensey, his choice for his landfall, lay only a point or two west of due north from St Valery. His boats were unusually small for even such limited sea travel as a one-way passage across the Channel and they were without any reserves of rowing power to pull them through even slight vagaries of weather. As is shown in the Tapestry, many of them were heavily loaded with men, horses, arms and supplies. These craft would be almost unmanageable in anything but an exactly favourable wind and a moderate sea, for in any other conditions they would be swung and driven wherever wind and weather dictated, their small steering oar useless. William had had one sharp lesson about Channel weather after he had set out from the estuary of the Dives. He now knew from hard experience that he dare not put his ships out to sea in any wind not blowing towards St Valery from due south at moderate speed, and this binding restriction goes far to explain why he had to wait so long for his chance to set sail for England.

It would have been out of character for this sober man to have hoped, during the months of frustration, that the longed-for wind would eventually be granted to him at probably the most propitious moment of the whole year. It is worth pondering again for a moment the astonishing list of favourable factors. William did not know about many of them until after he had gambled and won. Among them were : a gapingly empty Channel, an unguarded English coast, his enemy engaged over 250 miles to the north of Pevensey with many of his Housecarls dead or too severely wounded to be able to respond to another sudden call to action far to the south, his only other rival for the English throne defeated and dead, and a considerable portion of the native population (including the whipped and supine Earls Edwin and Morcar) either indifferent or hostile to their king. But on 27 September the one fact which filled William's mind was that the right wind was blowing for him at last and that he must be off, with the least possible delay.

Although William of Poitiers is so verbose and fawning towards William, and often deliberately misleading, his account of the start of the invasion from St Valery is probably sufficiently reliable to enable us to imagine fairly accurately what happened. The final loadings of the ships were probably accomplished during the early part of the day. The least manageable of the cargo would obviously be the knights' horses, and there has been much discussion as to how exactly they were brought aboard. A likely procedure would be to line up the boats allotted to them against a ramp so that at high tide the animals could be easily led aboard and made as comfortable as possible in their rather unstable new environment until it was time to go. It is likely that William led his fleet out of port as he stood upon the deck of his flagship *Mora* about the middle of the afternoon. He wanted to use several hours of daylight to get his fleet well out to sea before dusk. Sunset on that day is estimated to have occurred at 5.39 pm. The fleet would consequently have been able, in the long English twilight, to continue concerted movement until about 6.15 pm.

Since he could not count for sure upon the English coast near the important port of Hastings being totally undefended, William had to make plans to ensure that his ships should not run the risk of making landfall haphazardly and in small groups which could be overwhelmed by even a small defending force. Accordingly, ship's captains were ordered by William's heralds to keep as close as they could to the *Mora* after they had left St Valery; when night fell they were to rest at anchor until they saw a signal light from *Mora*'s mast. They should follow this light as it moved north and then, after dawn, re-assemble close to it for the rest of the journey to Pevensey. William was the kind of commander to make the most careful calculations about time, distances and the likely speed of his fleet in the current weather conditions. He probably kept his fleet moving for some hours in darkness behind his signal light, aiming to sail as near to Pevensey as could be managed so that dawn should find them so placed as to expose them to the shortest possible period of risk of being spotted and intercepted in daylight by any English warships which might still be in commission and on Channel patrol.

The chronicler records that all went well for William and his fleet during the first hours at sea but that dawn disclosed a most disconcerting situation to those aboard the *Mora*. 'In the morning an oarsman sent by the duke to the masthead was asked whether he could sight the following fleet but he replied that he could see nothing but sea and sky,' wrote William of Poitiers. The Duke

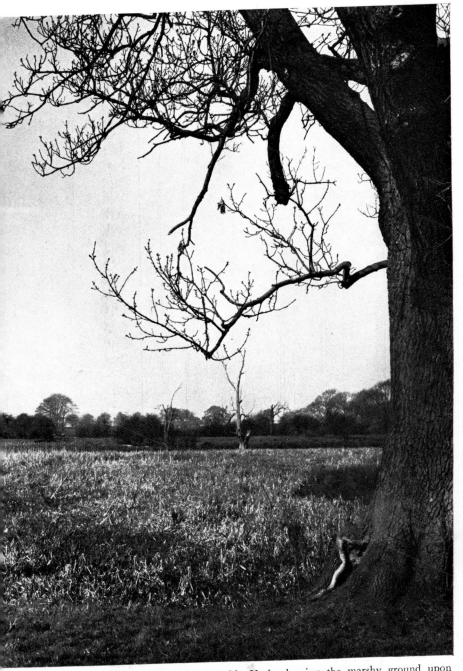

The battleground at Gate Fulford just outside York, showing the marshy ground upon which Harald Hardrada cornered the defending Northumbrians.

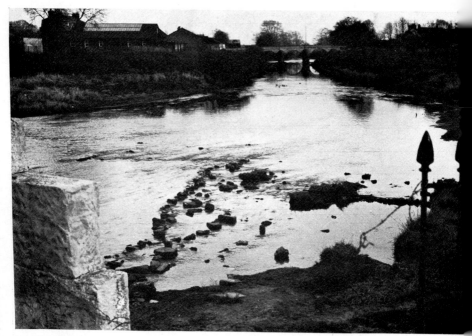

8 The point where King Harold and his Housecarls crossed the River Wharfe at Tadcas
Yorkshire, on their way to battle at Stamford Bridge.

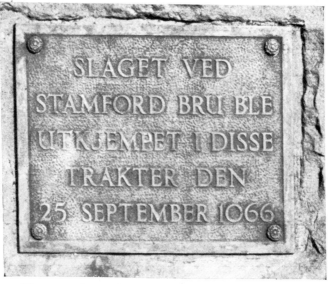

SLAGET VED
STAMFORD BRU BLE
UTKJEMPET I DISSE
TRAKTER DEN
25 SEPTEMBER 1066

9 The approximate site of the Battle of Stamford Bridge is
commemorated in Norwegian and English.

promptly ordered *Mora*'s anchor to be cast and, hiding whatever dismay he felt within, he put on a very good show indeed. To indicate that he was not at all discomfited by *Mora*'s loneliness, he ordered a large meal for himself and, says the scribe, 'accompanying it with a bumper of spiced wine he dined in good spirits as if he were in a room of his own house.' Presumably William was unlike many other renowned naval commanders who never went to sea without being seasick; and we hope that those of his companions who were similarly lucky were invited to share the large meal and the bumper of wine. After the shipboard feast William sent the seaman aloft for the second time. Now he saw four ships; and when he climbed the mast for the third time he cried out that 'the numberless masts clustered together looked like trees in a forest.' This was much better. Spirits soared again aboard the *Mora*. 'We leave it to the reader to judge how the confident hope of the duke was now turned to joy, and how from the depths of his heart he gave thanks to God for his mercy,' the chronicler adds unctuously.

It was good sailing for the fleet for the rest of the trip. Almost all the Norman ships put into a great star-shaped lagoon at Pevensey about 24 hours after they had left St Valery. This invasion, one of the most momentous in the history of the world, was also one of the quietest and smoothest. Troops and seamen beached their craft and stepped ashore without so much as one spear or hostile arrow to hinder them, without one English warrior challenging their descent upon his soil. But they did not go unseen. The port of Hastings had been founded long ago by a tribal family bearing its name. Now it occupied snugly a strip of shore line about ten miles east of Pevensey Lagoon and was a well-used Channel port. There can be no doubt that Englishmen watching from Hastings espied the great company of ships slowly looming inshore and, divining what was happening at last, despatched riders to London, 70 miles away to the north-north-east beyond the forests of the Andredsweald, to give the alarm to Harold's deputies. William knew about this, but also that he need not be too concerned about it, for pro-Norman informants would give him all the news about the Battle of Stamford Bridge and would assure him that Harold was almost 300 miles away. William had achieved the hoped-for miracle of an unopposed crossing and landing, and he could count now upon a welcome period of at least a week in which to consolidate his position at Pevensey and send his troops about in well-armed parties to seize

E

and plunder food and other stores in a large section of Sussex, before having to give a thought to molestation by Harold.

Only one mishap is recorded as having marred the perfection of William's landing. One or two of his boats lost touch with the rest of the fleet some time during the night and strayed far to the east to come ashore eventually at Romney, nearly 50 miles east of Pevensey. The men aboard the ships fared exactly as William had calculated would happen to his whole fleet if it lost cohesion. Romney was a fortified borough like Hastings and it had enough defenders, sailors as well as soldiers, to overcome parties of raiders, if not enough to resist a massive invasion such as William's. They effectively disposed of the luckless Normans, some of whom were probably too seasick to fight hard and all of whom were tired after a night and day at sea. All were slaughtered. Their doom was the more certain because they had had the ill fortune to stray upon a stretch of English coast which they should have avoided at all costs. The three Channel ports of Sandwich, Dover and Romney all maintained permanent defences independent of the national fyrd, on condition that each of them provided the king with 20 ships carrying crews of 21 apiece for two weeks' service at need per year. Sandwich, 13 miles to the north of Dover, was the chief land-sea terminal between England and northern Europe, at the end of a Roman road connecting London with Canterbury and the coast. William knew that this Kentish region would be defended even though Harold had had to disband the national forces, and for this reason alone he would never have chosen it for his landfall even if it had not lain much too far east from Normandy to suit him. The killing of his strayed troops by the defenders of Romney was an affront which William was not to forget. In due time, the town paid forfeit to him for what had been done.

William and Caesar

In thus invading Britain, William was doing approximately what Julius Caesar had done 1,120 years earlier, but he did it with far greater attention to detail and he reaped the appropriate rewards. The contrast between the planning and execution of the two invasions is highly enlightening with regard to the characters of two

of the most notable soldiers the world has ever seen – and the mighty
Caesar does not come off best by any means.

In 55 BC he resolved to make a reconnaissance in force of the
south-east coast of England as a preliminary to an invasion proper,
but he seems to have tackled the task in surprisingly slipshod
fashion. As a start, he sent over the Channel one of his officers,
Caius Volusenus, in a fast galley to assess the possibilities of a
landing at Dover. Apart from doing this, Caesar did not trouble to
find out much about either the terrain or the spirit of the Belgic
tribesmen whom he intended to dispossess. And Caius Volusenus
let him down badly by going back to Portius Itius (Boulogne) with
a verdict that Dover would be suitable for a landing. The man does
not seem to have noticed those high white cliffs for which Dover
has since become sentimentally renowned; perhaps it was a foggy
day.

Caesar duly put out from Portius Itius at midnight on 24–25
August with two Legions, the Seventh and Tenth, amounting to
8,000 men, plus supporting cavalry in 80 infantry barges and 18
horse transports. The cavalry is assumed to have sailed independently from Ambletouse, about 8 miles from Boulogne, but it never
reached Dover. Overtaken by a sudden storm, the horse transports,
carrying an unhandy and easily scared cargo, had to turn back.
Caesar and his legionaries were off Dover by 9 am to find the surf
unruly and uninviting to men accustomed to manoeuvring on dry
land; and the white cliffs were manned on top by tribesmen armed
with darts and other missiles. Wisely, Caesar gave an order for his
fleet to sheer off. The ships turned east to sail with the Channel
drift and came ashore on a stretch of beach at Deal, some ten miles
away, which had comparatively low ground behind it. Again, the
legionaries hesitated about wading ashore but inspired, as Caesar
himself relates, by the standard bearer of the Tenth Legion who
leapt into the waist-high water and dared the soldiers to be branded
with the ignominy of failing to follow their flag, the legionaries
then waded ashore. They were resisted by the Belgae, but experience
and discipline triumphed and the beachhead was secured. Caesar's
troubles were not yet over. He had neglected to learn about the
powerful effect of the moon upon tides in the narrow strait and on
the night of the full moon the sea flung his transports damagingly
against each other, and even some of his beached galleys were
smashed. To add to his frustration and anger, the horse transports

turned up at last on the fourth night of the raid, but once again the weather scattered them and they had to trail back to Gaul without one horse being landed.

Caesar had now had enough. His carpenters patched up some of his transports from the timbers of 12 which were beyond repair and as soon as the weather cleared, he and his legionaries went home. As another distinguished professional, Napoleon, commented many hundreds of years afterwards : 'It was a second class show.' ('C'était une opération de deuxième ordre.') And also, as a more recent professional, Major-General J. F. C. Fuller, remarked in 1965, it showed that 'instinctively Caesar was a gambler, a man over-apt to chance his luck.' One can scarcely imagine such a contrast as that between Julius Caesar, the gambling optimist, and William of Normandy, the deep-thinking planner.

A year later Caesar showed that he had learned some but not all the lessons of the ill-fated raid. This time he sailed from Portius Itius and Ambletouse in 600 newly-designed Channel boats as well as 200 of the earlier ones, with five Legions (20,000 men), 200 cavalry-men and their mounts, an assorted auxiliary force and ample bag-gage, seige materials and stores. Once again the Channel was fickle. During a night voyage on 21–22 July a strong tide edged his big fleet far to the east towards the North Sea and if he had not been able to use his legionaries as oarsmen he might have ended his trip on the dunes of the Belgian and Dutch coasts. Thanks to great efforts by his men he was able eventually to get his fleet ashore at almost the pre-arranged point between Sandwich and Sandown, and this time there was no opposition, for the same reason that enabled William to enjoy the same absence of interference – that local people perceived that they could not hope to resist such an immense force and went into hiding to watch developments and bide their time.

The Channel had yet one more ugly surprise in store for Caesar. He had pushed some 12 miles inland and was directing his legion-aries in their first skirmish with the reviving Belgae when a messenger came to him with word that a gale had blown up during the night and had piled his ships upon the beach, completely collapsing 40 of them and battering many more. One lesson he had not learned was that he must beach all his vessels if he did not wish to suffer from the vicious caprices of the English Channel. He now proceeded belatedly to do this. Breaking off his engagement with the natives, he brought his tired, long-suffering soldiers back to the beach and put them to work hauling the hundreds of heavy craft to safety. The task took them 12 days, including the digging of a deep trench around the grounded ships to give them extra protection from wind and water. Then he resumed his systematic subjugation of England.

In 1066 William avoided most of Caesar's setbacks because he had planned his invasion with such meticulous care. Instead of making a headlong dash across the narrowest part of the Channel to the nearest promising beach, he had chosen for his haven a sheltered and capacious lagoon in which the effects of winds and tides would scarcely be felt by his ships. He also landed in an area which he knew to be thinly-populated, rather than the busy neighbourhood of Dover, Deal and Sandwich which was comparatively well-settled because there was always much going on there in cross-Channel traffic. In fairness, it must be recognized that William did owe something to his Roman predecessor. The fort guarding the Pevensey lagoon was one of six put up along the coast by the Romans. They were at Reculver, Richborough, Dover, Lympne, Anderida (Pevensey) and Portchester (Portsmouth). Their purpose had been to house garrisons, which were held always at readiness to repel seaborne raiders and invaders by the officer in charge of coastal defence who was known as The Count of the Saxon Shore. The fort at Pevensey would have been a welcome point of last resort for William's men if they had been attacked soon after landing and driven back towards the sea. It stood in ten acres of ground and was circled by walls 30 feet high and over 12 feet thick – a formidable citadel once William had had time to restore the depredations of several centuries of Anglo-Saxon neglect.

Comparison between the performance of the two invaders of 54–55 BC and AD 1066 indicates that William was easily the better soldier. He did have advantages in that the Channel favoured him by apparently remaining docile long enough after giving him a smooth passage for him to consolidate his landing, and he did not have to meet any organized opposition from the natives within the peninsula. He must have ordered a most thorough inspection of the south coast of England to have found the ideal situation for landfall at Pevensey. Caesar emerges on the other hand as no planner at all, a man who sent one seemingly incompetent officer across the Channel on a quick trip to survey the beach at Dover, only to find when he got there that not only was the beach unsuitable for landing but was vulnerable to what amounted to the first example of bombing in known English history – by men hurling down missiles from the clifftops.

Finally, as we note how again and again William avoided mistakes made by Caesar, it seems obvious that the Norman knew about the Roman's story of his misadventures and profited therefrom. He could not read Caesar's word for himself, but his prelates and clerks knew their Latin and he could hear the story from them as he planned his own expedition.

The Landfall

We should now take up again the question of why William chose Pevensey for his landing. Surprisingly, this question does not seem to have been considered and properly answered for many centuries after the event, one reason being that the succession of historians and others who were fascinated by what happened in 1066 concentrated upon, and quarrelled continually about, the political conundrum of the Conquest rather than upon many of its other aspects. Analysis of why it happened where it did was obscured by the study of why it happened at all.

One aggravation is that, as with most of the missing or now-debatable circumstances of the enigma of Hastings, the matter of William's choice of Pevensey was obviously explicable for a long time after 1066, and nobody bothered either to set down the facts or otherwise relay them. Not until J. A. Williamson, the eminent British maritime authority, reported in 1959 the fruits of years of research on the history and changing geography of the English Channel did it become perfectly clear at last that William picked Pevensey most carefully after prolonged thought and with the use of those gifts of military insight and common-sense which made him such an outstanding and successful general. He perceived that Pevensey offered invaluable natural advantages to an attacker coming in from the sea and that its surrounding terrain faced a defender with severe handicaps. The critical fact which escaped adequate attention during and after the Middle Ages, when the study of the Conquest began to intensify, is that the outline and

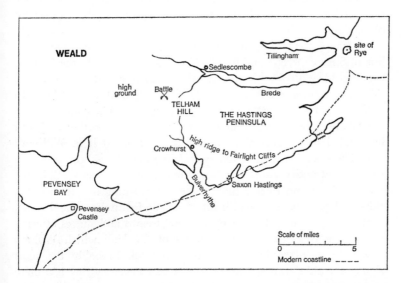

The Hastings coastline in the eleventh century. The shore-lines are shown as at high water.

physical characteristics of the southern English coastline had changed dramatically during the 400 or 500 years which had passed since the Battle of Hastings was fought.

By painstakingly reconstructing the features of the coastline from all surviving records and other evidence, Dr Williamson showed that the landing site at Pevensey was not only easily the most suitable between Portsmouth and Dover but that the immediate region of England to which it gave access was so well-contained – almost moated – that the only feasible entry into it from the hinterland, particularly the direction of London, by a defending army was on a very narrow saddle of ground to the north-east. This, as William accurately calculated, had to be exactly the route by which Harold and his troops must march upon him if they decided to attack him soon after his landing, instead of allowing him to languish during the winter. One decisive fact is thereby established : that the Battle of Hastings was fought on a field chosen by William. Further, as we shall see, the sequence of events between 28 September and 14 October abundantly proves the tragic truth that, by precipitately hurling himself and his army into an early battle so soon after the debilitating victory at Stamford Bridge and the forced rides up and down England, Harold fell into a deadly trap set by his enemy.

The map, p. 135, depicts a startling difference between the coast-line of Sussex in 1066 and today. The strongest winds in the English Channel have always blown from the south-west and the west, and their accumulative effect since the eleventh century has been to straighten out the coastline : pebbles, rocks and other material from the Channel bed have been thrust diagonally upon the land and have filled in most of the features which marked it in William's day. The coast between Pevensey and Rye must have been in Saxon times an attractive vista, seen from the sea, of large and small inlets, lagoons, bays and river estuaries. Relentless silting by innumerable tides and gales have turned it into a mostly featureless straight line, broken only here and there by narrow streams and sluices offering no facility whatever for manoeuvres of the kind which William was able to make in the autumn of 1066. Probably the most significant difference is that whereas today Pevensey Bay is a mere name, in 1066 it was a great tidal lagoon several miles wide at its seaward entrance and stretching some five miles inland.

On a tip of land marking the westerly entry into the lagoon stood the small Roman fort, probably falling into ruins. There was a difference of more than 20 feet between high and low tide in the lagoon. At low tide the lagoon was little more than an expanse of muddy marshland intersected by many runnels, and doubtless the home of snipe, wild duck and other water fowl. At high tide it was a deep and wide body of seawater lapping the walls of the fort and running into the furthermost inlets and swamps of the roughly star-shaped indentation of the shore line.

It obviously offered a magnificent landfall at high water, or soon thereafter, to an invasion fleet. Boats would be easily beached and very soon after grounding would be altogether out of the water. The lagoon had one other outstanding advantage in that it gave easy access – easy, that is to say, when there was no powerful defending fleet or land force to dispute passage – to a large contained peninsula, of which the established port of Hastings was the beating heart. The peninsula comprised about 50 square miles and went furthest inland on the site of the present town of Battle, seven miles north of Hastings. One highly desirable feature of the peninsula to William's eye was that at its northern boundary (at Battle) it

narrowed to a neck of land little more than a mile wide. This
bottleneck was the only practicable link between the peninsula and
the rest of England. Provided he kept it guarded he could feel
secure against being overrun without a fight. He could fortify his
encampment and ravage the homes and farms within the peninsula
to keep his forces fed and supplied for quite a while with forced
auxiliary labour, horses, cattle and whatever else offered. Given
enough time and luck, he *might* even make himself impregnable to
any assault which Harold or whoever else ruled England might
mount against him on that one narrow front to the north. But
this negative concept would not gain England for him. Sooner or
later he would have to lunge out of the peninsula and William
could by no means count on the fact that by the time he was
ready to do so, he would not have to face a defender who had
mobilized a superior force against him.

Now that he had landed safely and obtained a footing on such
favourable ground he could plan his immediate strategy on answers
to several questions which presented themselves. Had Harold disposed of the Norwegians or was Harald Hardrada to be his adversary in the struggle for England? If, as seemed most likely, Harold
was still king, how much support did he command inside his
kingdom? Could he be lured down to Pevensey for an early confrontation on William's terms? Or would he be clever enough to bide
his time, hoping to seal the invader within the peninsula while
he gathered his strength for a springtime frontal assault by land and
by a strengthened and remobilized fleet in the rear? This last was
a prospect which William could not ponder with comfort and he
must do everything he could to stave it off.

The map on p. 135 clearly traces the outline of the peninsula
within which, if William could manage it, all would soon be decided.
 Two miles east of the port of Hastings was another lagoon known
as Bulverhythe, nothing like the size of the Pevensey lagoon but
still a substantial inlet three miles wide at the coast and resembling
a two-pronged lake reaching several miles inland at high tide. It
sealed William's flank from attack from Hastings, for it was a far
more effective barrier than thousands of fighting men. It was fed
by a number of streams flowing from the western fringe of the
peninsula and it never went altogether dry – another useful characteristic. And there was an even more formidable barrier to continue
the protection of this flank closer to the north-eastern bounds of the

peninsula. This was yet another lagoon formed by the long, wide estuary of the river Brede. It penetrated as far inland as the hamlet of Sedlescombe, eight miles from the coast. Any commander seeking to assault William from the Kentish hinterland would certainly think twice about committing his men to an amphibious attack across the river Brede.

Such was the character of the area around Hastings, hard to imagine today, but still there in somewhat modified form in the sixteenth century, when tidal waters were flowing as far inland as Sedlescombe. They were flowing much more determinedly and widely 500 years earlier.

William Consolidates

Scribes writing many years after 1066, some of them over 100 years later, produced a variety of picturesque accounts of what happened immediately after William landed. Most of them are best regarded as fanciful and untrustworthy as a whole, but probably founded upon a few fundamental true facts. There seems to be no doubt, for example, that one of the first moves William made was to secure himself from any surprise attack from the sea or by land from defenders placed within the peninsula itself, who were not dependent for help and reinforcement from outside. The principal point of danger here was Hastings itself. So William moved promptly to seize it. He sent forces to take it by land from the lagoon at Pevensey, probably via Crowhurst. In advancing upon Hastings they would be automatically enlarging the territory he controlled. He also sent men by sea along the coast and via the mouth of the smaller lagoon at Bulverhythe. Although fortified and guarded by a local garrison, Hastings would be in no situation to make much show of resistance to the strong contingents William could send against them. There is, in fact, no word anywhere to suggest that Hastings made even a token defence. The Anglo-Saxon Chronicle, which could be expected to record any such skirmish, says simply: 'As soon as his men were fit for service, they constructed a castle at Hastings.' It sounds very much as if William's men simply took over Hastings and did what they wished there.

It had become almost instinctive by this period for Normans to build a castle as a defensive stronghold. Judging by drawings in the Tapestry and other enduring illustrations, these rough-and-ready creations were made of whatever wood was easily available; they were not intended to be permanent but to serve as a home and fortress for troops engaged on a campaign. They were usually built on a hill or rising ground and were protected by a drawbridge to cut off entry by an attacking force. The permanent Norman castle came later. The tactical purpose of the castle built at Hastings was apparently the usual one, but it also had a specific dual purpose. From its top rampart, or maybe even a tower, sentinels could give early warning of the coming of a hostile force either by sea or land. It could also serve as a rallying point for William's soldiers if, by some unforeseen chance, Harold was able to pounce suddenly upon them. They could hold out against him from within it for a long time, long enough for reinforcements to reach the spot and make a counter-attack to break the siege. While the castle was being built William sent other men all over the peninsula to plunder, to seize able-bodied men and women to work as serfs for the invaders, and to spread the grim word far afield that William was the new master of Sussex and intended to remain so. As usual, William acted without mercy. His men were told to burn and pillage without pity, and the thoroughness with which they obeyed him was confirmed 20 years later by entries in the Domesday Book survey of England which described once-viable settlements in and even beyond the limits of the peninsula starkly as 'wasta'. Among the *vils* which the Normans are known to have ravished were: Ashburnham, Bexhill, Crowhurst, Hurstmonceux, Ninfield, Pevensey, Sedlescombe and Whatlington. Others named in the Domesday Survey cannot be identified, for the pitiful reason that they were so thoroughly despoiled that they were never rebuilt.

There was, as ever, purpose as well as ruthlessness behind William's tactics. He wanted news of the havoc he was making in Harold's own former earldom to reach the King quickly. He knew Harold's impetuous nature and intended to lure him down to Hastings as soon as possible, so that he could be brought to battle. He must be defeated soon, in case the whole of England might after all fall in behind him and confront the invader with superior strength. And of course William particularly wanted to force Harold to face him on the narrow strip of land north of Pevensey and Hastings. Here he could bring into more concentrated action his squadrons of cavalry on a limited front from which their prey could only escape by turning tail and running, thereby exposing themselves to being cut down by their mounted pursuers.

While consolidating his position, and probably having at least some reinforcements and supplies ferried to him across the Channel when the weather allowed, as well as flinging out bait to attract his enemy into his clutches, William was also gaining intelligence.

His scribes have written elaborate accounts of how Norman nobles living in south-east England hurried to see William to tell him all the news he did not know. While the tales are overdrawn and biassed, the fact that the writers were able to name some of the informants does give some substance to their stories and warrants an assumption that William was well and quickly supplied with information to help him decide on his immediate policy. About a week after he had landed at Pevensey he knew that Harald Hardrada had been bloodily wiped out of contention for the English throne and that Harold, somewhere in the northcountry, had heard of the Norman invasion and the ravishing of the peninsula. Thus, William knew that he must prepare with all speed to meet, and beat, Harold soon if his estimate of his enemy's character was well founded. One of William's best informants on such matters was apparently Robert Fitzwymark, an Anglo-Norman who was related to William on his mother's side and was close to the English court. Fitzwymark had been one of Edward the Confessor's aristocratic Norman friends. He was also one of those men who throughout history are to be found close to the seat of power but who do not seek direct power for themselves. They survive reigns, revolutions and other passing upheavals to die eventually of old age. Robert is shown in the Bayeux Tapestry among the small company of elite at Edward's deathbed on 5 January 1066. Harold is seen standing close to him, indicating that they were not open enemies. According to the chroniclers, Robert's advice to William was that since Harold had crushed the Norwegian interloper and his own brother 'and hastens towards you at the head of innumerable troops all well equipped for war and against whom your own warriors will prove of no more account than a pack of curs,' William as a wise man should not offer battle immediately but stay behind his entrenchments and build up his forces in security. Although this advice was spurned it was evidently appreciated, for after the Conquest William appointed Robert Fitzwymark Sheriff of Essex and never turned against him.

Fitzwymark's information about Harold's move south to confront William was sound enough. Harold had left York for London by 1 October with all his Housecarls fit for service plus, almost certainly, a number of northern volunteers willing to join him in protecting his kingdom. There could not have been many such men. If, as we know, northern and southern England were still cool to each other, divided by economic and other rivalries until the early days of the twentieth century (and even today), they must have been like two different countries in Harold's time. This is inferentially confirmed by the fact that, as far as we know, Edward the Confessor never set foot in the north of England and Harold only went there in emergency – once to head off a brewing rebellion soon after he had been crowned and once again to confront Hardrada.

Harold's feat in leading his Housecarls on a memorable ride from York to London demonstrated again his surpassing resilience and military agility. He appeared in London so soon after the Battle of Stamford Bridge that it seems scarcely believable that he was still in York when he heard of William's landing. Yet that is a firm tradition which has persisted since the eleventh century and although it is unsupported by any firm evidence it could be true. On the other hand, the timetable of the fantastic surge of history during the month of October 1066 is certainly more comprehensible if it is conceded that Harold was already on his way south, when messengers intercepted him with the news from Pevensey. Why should he not have been making for London by 1 October? He needed urgently to be back there, quite apart from any knowledge of William's arrival. He had been in only insecure control of the south of England – then, as now, the heart of the country – when he had had to ride north to destroy Hardrada. Anything could have happened in London while he had been away and he would have learned very little about it. He had left the south coast gapingly bare of defenders. He needed to start immediately on the task of rebuilding his crippled and mostly demobilized fleet and to remuster the militia while there was still time for William to invade. As a measure of long-term strategy, he must set about building up all the defences of England against a certain invasion in the spring of 1067 if William was held back until then. Above all,

Harold had to use every means available to him to bring the whole of England under his royal banner.

There was now no need to stay in the north, for he had confirmed his authority there by the surest method of all – devastating victory in battle. He need fear neither further insurrection in Yorkshire and the whole of Northumbria nor any new invasion from Scandinavia. Even Malcolm of Scotland would now be quiet for a while. Why then linger in York? A convincing circumstantial case may be made to support a theory that he turned for the south again within two or three days of the Battle of Stamford Bridge, perhaps even by coincidence on the very same day (28 September) that William was leading his fleet into Pevensey Lagoon. We face no hard contradiction of such an assumption. Harold's movements during the ten days or so between the battle on 25 September and his arrival in London were never formally recorded at the time and have never been even partly confirmed. The only certain fact is that he was in London by 5 October. He probably did not try to have all his Housecarls and his other soldiers in the capital by that date. It is more likely that he and a select company of his men rode hard to establish a presence in London, while the rest of his army followed at a more leisurely pace to cover between 30 and 35 miles a day, using pauses on the journey to recruit and to stir support, if not enthusiasm, for his cause. Harold had a great need to gather new troops by immediate enlistment to back him up in facing the Normans : It is, therefore, reasonable to envisage his men making stops all the way through Mercia and the south central shires to spread the glowing news of Harold's triumph at Stamford Bridge and to impress upon thegns and peasants in the towns and settlements his need for fighting men to preserve the kingdom from yet another outsider.

The likely picture, then, is of Harold and his bodyguard riding pell mell for London along unkept Roman roads, by forest tracks, and through clusters of farms and homesteads. Other Housecarls ride more slowly after them, stopping to propagandize and recruit. The foot soldiers, recruits, camp followers and others follow at whatever speed they can manage. They probably marched an average of 20 miles a days and so would all have been with Harold again in London by 9 or 10 October, at the latest. This is purely theoretical reconstruction but it does fit perfectly with the few established facts about Harold's movements until the Battle of

Hastings. And it seems to make common-sense out of an abundance
of disparate medieval assertions, believable and otherwise.

Harold spent about five days after he reached London in
attending to outstanding administrative affairs and gathering
strength for the coming ordeal. He had obviously made up his
mind what he was going to do. Ample evidence is available (and will
be quoted later) to indicate that Harold resolved to hasten towards
the coast as swiftly as he could. There he would set his army firmly
along the ridge across the Hastings-Pevensey peninsula, thus bottling
up his enemy and blocking any egress by William from the peninsula. He would keep William penned up there until he withered
from lack of sustenance or until Harold built up enough strength
to send an army swarming down from the ridge while William's rear
was assailed by an English fleet. Harold's strategy was based on
a close knowledge of the terrain involved. It was part of his own
original earldom – and the people within the peninsula who were
terrorized by William were his own people. He had passed much
of his early life on the south coast and its hinterland. He had a
manor at Bosham, some 60 miles west of the peninsula, and owned
several other homes in Sussex and Kent. He knew all about the
rivers and ravines enclosing the peninsula, and he certainly knew
the ridge guarding its northern boundary, for the only road or, more
properly, the track between London and Hastings crossed the ridge.

Harold must have calculated that it would be easy to man this
front with even a small army, for it was one of only about 1,000
yards. He could not have foreseen much difficulty in keeping the
invaders locked up in the peninsula until the fogs and damps of an
English winter put an end to any but routine military effort; the
winter respite could only add to Harold's advantage. It did not
work out thus for Harold. He seems to have greatly under-estimated
the size and striking power of William's infantry and cavalry
and, perhaps more important, William's boldness in military
offensiveness. He obviously did not believe it possible for William
to have brought a force across the water powerful enough to make
an immediate challenge to even the depleted army now at Harold's
disposal.

One looks vainly for alternative explanations of Harold's moves
and tactics. It simply will not suffice to argue that he careered
down the length of England and hurled himself against William
simply because his heart was bleeding for the sufferings of the

comparatively few people overrun by William in the peninsula. William was correct in estimating that Harold was impetuous; but he was not *that* impetuous. Nor was he a raw military amateur, all impulse and no judgement. To the extent that he reacted instantly to meet the invasion, he took William's bait – but not for the reason which William had imagined. He took it believing he had William's measure, and he was proved wrong. His tactics seemed sound enough – until he was outmanoeuvred by a sharper and more adventurous adversary than he had expected. His miscalculations brought him a warrior's death and changed England's destiny.

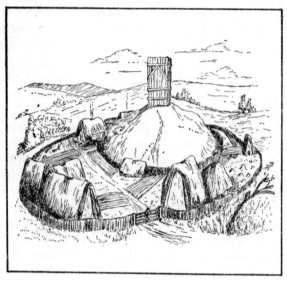

A Saxon *vil*. Drawing by Joyce Palmer.

8

Harold's Last Ride

Having decided on a course of action, Harold moved with the
utmost energy to fulfil it. He was in a hurry, again, as the pressures
which beset this unlucky king from the moment of his coronation
tightened. The Saxon chroniclers in Abingdon and Worcester were
by no means over-stating their case in recording that Harold 'was
not to enjoy a tranquil reign while he ruled the kingdom.' They
would have been closer to the truth if they had said that he was
granted scarcely a moment of tranquillity during the 40 weeks
and one day that he was on the throne of England.

The pressure upon him now was the need to get his army down
to the coast as quickly as he could. To achieve his decided
purpose, he must seal the Pevensey Peninsula before William could
forestall him. Encouraged by absence of opposition and strengthened
by reinforcements of men who would be eager to join him now
that he had so spectacularly overcome his first and biggest hazard
by landing unopposed and virtually without loss, William might
well advance over the undefended ridge and fan out over Wessex
and the rest of the south-east. He would then be hard to catch.
Harold had also to calculate that a swift effort against the invader
would keep and perhaps increase his authority over his people,
besides heartening those who were already being plundered and
enslaved or were in growing danger of such afflictions.

Five days was about the shortest imaginable period in which
Harold could prepare his counterstroke in London. The column
of marchers from York had to be given time to reach London
and there restore themselves before being asked to undertake yet
another forced march; the thegns and conscripted men of the fyrd
and the straggles of volunteers from the shires of the south
midlands had to be marshalled and drilled into some kind of
usable military condition; the armies of Gyrth and Leofwin,

Harold's brothers, had to be assembled in London. There were also all the innumerable chores of planning, housekeeping, arming to be accomplished, and arrangements made for the administration of the country while the king and many of his principal officers were away. London must have been a place of turmoil – excitement, anxiety, feverish industry, rumours, and open and furtive espionage – between 5 and 10 October. The city would be convulsed by its first experience as the *de facto* capital of England coping with an unparalleled national emergency. It was still quite a small and rural-looking settlement compared with the older and more mature cities of the world such as Rome, Alexandria and Byzantium, even though it now had the new building of wood which was to grow into Westminster Abbey, one of the most august monuments to Christianity the world was ever to see. Harold's use of London as the closest base to the point of his present danger confirmed its eclipse of Winchester as the heart of England.

One worry must have nagged even such a sanguine man as Harold. We know from entries in the Chronicle and from other documents that the response to his hurried call to arms was ominously meagre. He simply had not had time to send out his agents across the country on a systematic recruiting campaign, or go out himself to bestir Englishmen into joining him against the foreign invader. He had perforce to make do, for the time being, with whatever forces he could gather immediately, or let William over-run the south. It is certain from entries in the Domesday Book that men from Berkshire, Hampshire and as far distant as Hunting-don, Cambridge and Leicestershire rallied to Harold's side, and several abbots and priors were among the militant churchmen who led small contingents into his army. Among these was Aelfwig. abbot of the New Minster of Winchester, who fought for Harold at the head of 12 men and, with them, perished at Hastings. Because this elderly cleric had been a member of the House of Godwin and had so flagrantly opposed William in battle, part of the New Minster was later confiscated and many of its rights and privileges extinguished. Another fighting clergyman was Leofric, Abbot of Peterborough, who was so severely wounded at Hastings that he died 18 days later, having staggered away from the battlefield probably while the fighting was still going on, and somehow made his way back to his monastery 150 miles away to the north.

There are also records showing that some other notable Anglo-Saxons were effectively loyal to Harold and fought alongside him, but they are few. Two Englishmen who did so, at the cost of their lives, are perpetuated in the Chronicles of Abingdon Monastery in Berkshire. One was Thurkill (or Turchill) who held lands at Kingston Bagpuize, now a lovely Thames-side hamlet and the site of a picturesque old river ferry close to Abingdon. The other was Godric, who held the office of Sheriff of Fyfield, a village between Kingston Bagpuize and Abingdon. Godric's wife had been a personal attendant to Edward the Confessor. This is confirmed by an entry in the Domesday survey that his wife held land in Berkshire which had been given to her by Edward as a reward from the king for looking after his dogs at Abingdon. They were presumably hounds he used from time to time for hunting, the one sport of which he was, surprisingly in view of his distinctive mildness, very fond.

The lands of both these men were seized after Hastings by Henry de Ferrières, although Thurkill's were the property of the Abbey and those of Godric had been held on a lease 'of three lifetimes' from the same institution. De Ferrières would hardly have made the seizures without the approval of Duke William. He may even have been fulfilling William's policy of taking stern forfeit for opposition to him on the field of Hastings. It is illuminating to read a writ sent by William to Baldwin, Abbot of Bury St Edmunds, some years after the battle, ordering that the Abbot should 'hand to me all the land which those men held who belonged to St Edmund's soke [area of jurisdiction] and who stood in battle against me and there were slain.' In the same document William confirmed that other tenants who had not fought him were now to be recognized as being in the care of the Abbot and 'I will not allow anyone to take from him anything I have given him.'

Thurkills (or Thirkells) were still living in Abingdon 907 years after the battle. Gordon Wilson Thirkell moved from one end of the town to the other in 1973 when he exchanged landlordship of The Broad Face public house for that of The Crown. He has no inkling of the twists and turns in the skein of relationship with the Thurkill who fought and fell at Hastings, but he is proud to think that such a relationship exists.

No doubt Harold's own subjects in Wessex, comprising a substantial stretch of comparatively well-populated country which was uncomfortably threatened from William's beachhead, joined him out of an acute sense of self-interest as well as from loyalty to their kingly earl. But there was neither time nor, probably, enthusiasm for a substantial answer to Harold's defending summons in the regions away to the west and north-west – Dorset, Devon, Cornwall, Somerset, Gloucester, Worcester, Hereford and the north midlands as far as Manchester. One recalls that 15 years earlier the people of Somerset had fought to stop Harold from returning into England from his banishment by Edward the Confessor; and the thinly-peopled and remote areas of the north-west to the vague Scottish border would not even know what was going on in London and the south. There is no evidence of the existence of any sizeable settlements north-west of Lancaster in the eleventh century. Unlike the vigorous north-east, founded principally by invading Vikings who were Harold's forbears, the region seems to have been a forested wilderness giving shelter and sustenance more to animals than men, and scarcely to be considered in any sense but geographically as part of the kingdom. The Romans had found the thin civilization of Cumberland, for example, to have been culturally at the level of the Bronze Age and they used the area almost exclusively for camps, way stations, and communications. In the tenth century King Edmund Ironsides valued the territory so lightly that he gave the settlement of Carlisle and a considerable surrounding region of Cumberland to Malcolm of Scotland. It was an unhappy day for Carlisle, since its people were to know little peace for the next seven centuries and were to receive scant help or sympathy from government in Westminster. The attitude of the more populous county of Lancashire in the eleventh century may be deduced from its state of mind early in the twentieth century. Even then there was suspicion of, and often hostility to, the national government in London and some proud local spirits preferred, perhaps only half seriously though none the less significantly, to toast their king by his closer title of 'Duke of Lancaster'. The predecessors of such stalwarts would not have had much time to spare for a half-Danish king hailing from the distant south of England.

Harold is also reported to have ordered the refitting of his demobilized and battered fleet still clustered in the Thames estuary and to have told its captains to sail southwards as soon as they could via Sheerness, the North Foreland and the Straits of Dover, to be in position to fall upon William should he be forced to try to return to Normandy. Alternatively, they were to try to intercept any sea-borne reinforcements coming across the Channel from Normandy. He also had under his control, of course, the remnants of Hardrada's invasion fleet. It is to be assumed that during the week of 1–8 October some at least of these ships would have been made operable and have reached the south, along with some of the ships of that small fleet of Morcar's which had not fought in September but had exerted its tactical pressure in the Ouse and the Wharfe, in the manner of so many fleets in history.

Worried and disappointed as Harold must have been at the slowness and smallness of his mobilization against the growing danger, he seems to have decided by Tuesday, 10 October, that he was now strong enough to man the critical ridge north of Pevensey and that, in any case, he dare not wait any longer before setting out for it. On that day or the following (Wednesday) morning he left London with every Housecarl and warrior who could be found a horse, and set out for the coast of Sussex, leaving word in London and at every settlement through which he and his men rode that all the 'foot-sloggers' should follow him as swiftly as they could. He must have picked up more strength as he rode through his own earldom, and by the time he and his mounted force emerged from the Andredsweald, an enormous area of mostly oak forest covering east Sussex, and entered the undulating approaches to the coast near Sedlescombe, he may have been feeling more comfortable.

Provided his theory was well-founded that William did not yet have enough strength to burst out of the peninsula and attack him, time would be working for him. With the beachhead sealed off he could decide his future tactics according to how various elements in the military equation developed – the weather, how William's own situation fared for good or ill, and the progress Harold made in massing the manpower of much of England behind him. On these factors would obviously depend Harold's next move – an attack upon William before November or a winter siege of the peninsula. Unfortunately, all hinged on the accuracy of his assessment of William's situation and thinking.

Harold rode out of London at the head of his mounted House-carls by way of Tabard Street, which from very early times had been the only serviceable exit to the south, and headed thence via the Roman highway of Watling Street as far as Rochester and Chatham. Like most other Roman roads Watling Street had been built with admirable thoroughness on a ridge varying from four to eight feet in height according to the undulations in the terrain through which it passed. Part of it was exposed at a depth of 8 feet 6 inches during excavations at Strood, outside Rochester, in 1897, when its outstandingly substantial composition was revealed. According to Thomas Codrington, the authority on Roman roads, it had a foundation 3 feet 6 inches thick of timber, Roman tiles and other materials. This was topped by five inches of rammed chalk, seven inches of finely broken flint, and nine inches of small pebble gravel mixed with black earth. On top of all this was a paved surface between six and eight inches thick. The track was 14 feet wide and provided plenty of room for horsemen to pass pedestrians plodding along it.

As long as the Romans were caring for such thoroughfares they were maintained in good condition but most of them, including Watling Street, are believed to have been grossly neglected after the Roman dominion over England disintegrated. This notwithstanding, Harold and his men must have been able to make good time on such a soundly-made road. Passing along it through the settlement of Rochester, still sometimes called in the eleventh century by its original Roman name of Durobrivae, they swung off it to the right at the top of Chatham Hill to take another minor Roman road or track to Maidstone. Then, this long and hard-riding column of fit and disciplined fighting men had to pick its way at a somewhat slower pace along rough tracks through the densities of the Andredsweald, one of the country's great forests. The Andredsweald, known to the early Saxons as Andreds Leag and apparently named in honour of some long-forgotten figure, is estimated to have covered well over 100 miles from east to west roughly between Folkstone and Southampton, and to have been an average of 40 miles deep from north to south. The region which it clothed with trees, mostly oak, is still well-wooded although the weald as an entity has gone, erased by the needs of industry, agriculture and housing as the kingdom has developed. Today it survives residually in the Ashdown and Tilgate forests and various other smaller woodlands. Much of the rest of the forest was devoured through the Middle Ages by the iron and glass industries and the use of its timber to build the Royal Navy.

No record was made of the exact route which Harold took through the Andredsweald but there is evidence to suggest that he and his troops emerged from it somewhere just north of the present village of Sedlescombe. Local historical records show that in 1876 a decayed wooden box which was almost certainly a Saxon army pay chest was unearthed just off the Roman road running through Sedlescombe at a point some yards behind the village hall. In it were more than 1,000 coins of the reign of Edward the Confessor. This king's coins were of course still being widely used during Harold's brief reign and the inference may be made, with some justification, that the chest is a relic of Harold's last ride.

Passing through Sedlescombe, Harold made for the rallying point he had chosen for his army. It was nine miles north of the coast at Hastings and was on Caldbeck Hill, an eminence some 300 feet above Channel level. It is described rather romantically in the Anglo-Saxon Chronicle as 'The Hoar Apple Tree'. The choice of a tree as a rallying point for an army may sound odd to modern ears but we must appreciate that in the rural and only sparsely developed countryside of the eleventh century, a big tree, especially one standing alone in a clearing on a hill, was a land-mark known to everybody for many miles around and was easily identifiable by strangers coming from afar. Further, and this makes the choice of the landmark even more explicable, the spot where many historians believe the Hoar Apple Tree to have stood in 1066 was a junction point for several tracks coming from east and west and it was on Caldbeck Hill that the boundaries of three districts – Baldeslow, Ninfield, Hailesaltede – met. It is moving, exciting indeed, for a person of the twentieth century to stand on the gentle slopes of Caldbeck Hill and, feeling the breeze brushing the face, receive with its noiseless impact the imagined sounds of events in the second week of October so long ago – the clatter of iron-armed riders and walkers, the shouts of command, the ribaldry and the forced humour, the neighing of ponies whose senses tell them that once again danger lies ahead as an army gathers.

One final point emphasizes that Harold was following a common practice in choosing a tree as his rallying point. Archeologists have traced 14 references to a 'Hoar Apple Tree' as denoting a boundary and otherwise serving as a landmark in documents of Saxon Eng-land; and almost 200 years before the Battle of Hastings a tree served as a military mustering point and the actual site of combat.

The Battle of Assandune (Ashdown), three miles north of Lambourne in Berkshire, in 871, when Alfred the Great routed the Viking invaders of Wessex, was fought round 'a single thorn tree'. In the Domesday Survey over two centuries later one of the districts in Berkshire is described as Nachededorn (Naked Thorn). It contained the manor of the same name and also the manor of Ashdown.

Harold and his men are assumed to have reached The Hoar Apple Tree some time during Thursday, 12 October. There they rested from their ride of between 50 and 60 miles from London and are presumed to have been joined overnight by the first groups of auxiliaries, thegns and soldiers who had managed to get horses, as well as by other volunteers and conscripts responding to Harold's call to arms from the areas closest at hand. Then, next morning, Harold began despatching his growing army from Caldbeck Hill to the northern ridge of the peninsula. It was Friday, 13 October. The superstitious will instantly note the unlucky combination of day and date and draw the appropriate gloomy conclusions.

The distance from rallying point to ridge was little more than a mile and the way led mostly along the Hastings–London track. Once again, as we picture these armed men riding or trudging along that mile of track to the ridge overlooking a mildly sloping meadow, do the circumstances proclaim the certainty that neither they nor Harold had any thought of launching themselves against William within a matter of hours. They were really in no condition to do so. They had only just arrived in the area. They were expecting more and more men to join them during the next two or three days, not in a few hours. Their enemy was nowhere near them; he was several miles away and dispersed about the peninsula. They needed time to establish themselves firmly along the ridge and perhaps to build some obstacles and fortifications to protect them from a sudden attack. They were manning the ridge, then, as a blocking force. A prudent and seasoned general, Harold was placing them there as soon as possible because he wished to make sure that William's troops did not sneak out of the peninsula while the only exit was still open; the very presence of his Housecarls on the ridge, unprepared for battle as they were, would be enough (Harold calculated) to prevent that. So why on earth should he provoke battle before he was ready? According to one chronicler, only one-third of his total expected army was with him that Friday.

Other reporters confirm the nature of the disaster which was already looming before Harold as his men took up their positions less than 24 hours before it happened. A monk in Worcester wrote : 'William came upon him unexpectedly before his army was set in order.' Another monk wrote to the same effect in the Peterborough edition of the Chronicle when he related that William attacked Harold 'before all his host came up'. The evidence of these contemporary scribes in disclosing Harold's faulty judgement and William's bold opportunism is conclusive.

As the phenomenal importance of events in the autumn of 1066 became apparent in the twelfth and succeeding centuries, storytellers grasped the opportunity presented. Using their imaginations to add excitement to the drama, and often seeking to offer their own explanations of the enigma created by absence of proven facts, they seem to have invented events which simply did not happen. Thus, they said that messages passed between Harold and William during the second week of October 1066, and some even gave their versions of the substance of the threats, challenges, offers and counter-offers made by messengers on behalf of the two principals. They were relying on an assumption that a fairly common practice of pre-battle parleying was followed here. This could have been so, but since there is not one contemporary suggestion that such a thing happened and there is strong circumstantial evidence that it did not, we shall do well to set aside the tales of these latter-day scribes.

There was actually very little scope for exchanges since for most of the time between 28 September and 14 October the antagonists were hundreds of miles apart and, except during the last 12 night-time hours before the battle, one scarcely knew where the other was. Harold was almost continuously on the move between the Battle of Stamford Bridge and his arrival on the ridge above Hastings;* and during the period of five days when he was comparatively stationary in London from 5–10 October, there would scarcely have been time for more than one round trip by a messenger from

* The ridge and the battle area have become widely known as Senlac since 1066. The word is apparently based on a mention in local records of Battle Abbey of a tract of land called Santlache. This is probably the name by which the site of the Battle of Hastings became known after the Conquest. Bulwer Lytton used his novelist's imagination to suggest that the battle-field was called Sanguelac (Lake of Blood, very approximately).

William to Harold, or vice versa. One further important point must be considered. In all probability, one of the last things Harold wished to do was to give away either his location or his plans to William, for the essence of his reaction to the invasion was a resolve to make use of the element of surprise in his arrival at Hastings. There *might* have been some contact late on Friday, 13 October, but it is unlikely, for William, having resolved to seize the initiative by attacking Harold the next morning, would scarcely wish to give away anything about his plan in the few hours before he carried it out. Any such message he did send could only have been intended to mislead.

William seems to have recovered quickly from the surprise caused by the unexpected appearance of Harold's mustering army at the Hoar Apple Tree and on the ridge. That he *was* surprised is evident from statements which there is no reason to disbelieve that on the Friday many of his men were out foraging and pillaging and had to be hastily rounded up and directed back to base to get themselves ready to do what William quickly decided – to attack Harold as soon as possible after dawn next day. William obviously saw clearly that in the new situation created by Harold's arrival, it was for him a case of conquest now or probably never. His scouts and spies must have been keeping watch on the English from the moment that activity was noticed in the neighbourhood of the apple tree on Caldbeck Hill. William would know that when, rather late on the Friday, Harold began sending his men across the meadows of Caldbeck to Senlac, his enemy was as yet by no means at full strength but would be growing stronger almost by the hour as more and more men reached the rendezvous. At all costs, whatever the odds, William saw that he must assault and destroy Harold without delay, before those odds became too formidable.

There was one other strictly military consideration which William had to take into account. Harold must not be given time to settle down on Senlac ridge – to 'dig in', so to speak. As William pondered his situation on the Friday evening he had to recognize that one of his disadvantages next day would be in having to attack uphill towards the ridge and on a very narrow front giving scant opportunity for manoeuvre. Therefore, his best chance of victory lay in exploiting his bowmen and cavalry (both of which, he knew, Harold lacked) in skilful co-ordination. Harold must on no account be given time and opportunity to protect himself from either of them. He could do so, however, in two ways if he were given even one day's respite from attack. He could get his men to build a substantial wooden stockade along the ridge, behind which his army would crouch to avoid the showers of arrows which would precede an assault firstly by strongly armed infantry and then by the knights on horseback. He could also dig a ditch in front of the stockade to make the final approach difficult for both infantry and cavalry. If properly carried out, these defences could make Harold's troops close to invulnerable. Here therefore was another over-riding reason for William's decision to attack without delay.

A curious circumstance which confronts the inquirer into the enigma of Hastings is that one chronicler alone, among the many who in the eleventh and twelfth centuries wrote their versions of the encounter, states that Harold's men did in fact put up a fence of plaited and interlaced woodwork in front of them, in the few hours available before the Norman assault. He is Robert Wace, at one time a priest at Caen, in Normandy. But he was writing 90 years after the battle and his *Roman de Rou* is notable more for its appeal as a smoothly-written but fancy tale than for its reliability as evidence. The rhymed passage in which his description of the protective palisade occurs runs thus in translation from the Old French : 'They made in front of them shields of wattled ash and other woods; they raised these in front of themselves like hurdles joined and set close; they left no opening in them but made them into an enclosure.' Wace is hazy and not very convincing in his description. His claim has been almost unanimously dismissed by historians, rightly as one must conclude, for many reasons. It is felt that since he was writing so long after the battle he could very well have been confused by earlier references to old and abandoned fortifications and various gullies and ditches in front of and behind the English position on the ridge. Furthermore, there was not time between Harold's occupation of the Senlac position and the onset of battle for anything like a worthwhile palisade to have been built. Also, none of the contemporary or early Norman scribes says a word about any such palisade and the Bayeux Tapestry – which could certainly be expected to take any opportunity of magnifying William's victory over the odds against him – depicts the battle most clearly as happening upon open ground. Finally, there is also total unanimity among the chroniclers in their descriptions of Harold's army as being ranged in tight and thick formation behind a wall made of its own shields and nothing else. Perhaps Wace knew enough about military matters to perceive how vital it was for Harold to protect his line with a palisade if he possibly could and carelessly took it for granted that he actually managed to do this.

While Wace apparently imagined the English working furiously long after night had fallen on 13 October on the construction of a palisade, John Milton saw them very differently occupied. He is once again unfair to the England and the Englishmen of 1066. Writing some 600 years later in his history of the country he repeats a Norman calumny that during the night 'both sides prepared to fight the next morning, the English from singing and drinking all night, the Normans from confession of their sins and Communion of the Host.' Milton was allowing his evangelical obsessions to overcome his common-sense, for what he writes is simply unbelievable. The English must have been close to exhaustion after what they had been doing since they left London, and one imagines that the last thing most of them would seek would be an all-night carousal.

The more likely truth is that after having sent some of his troops, perhaps a thousand, to man Senlac ridge late in the day, Harold received the jarring news from scouts and spies that he had guessed wrongly. Far from skulking supinely close to his bases at Hastings and Pevensey on the coast, William was massing to attack him next day. Tired as Harold must have been after the frantic rushes of the past two weeks, and dispirited by the disturbing news he now had of imminent battle, he had nonetheless to make ready for the ordeal at hand. In all probability, he did so by sending as many men as he could muster to join the holding force already in position on Senlac ridge. They would improve their defences as much as possible before slumping down, dog tired, to take whatever rest they could before standing to arms in the morning and staking their lives against the invading Normans.

The Two Armies

We now come to the final critical aspect of the coming grapple between Harold and William. What were their relative strengths in manpower as they assembled to face each other? One assumption to be made with confidence is that William, besides being stronger than Harold had imagined, actually had more men under his command than Harold, although not necessarily more available for use as warriors in the field. Some evidence confirming his superior total strength is offered by the references in the Anglo-Saxon Chronicle, already quoted, to Harold's unpreparedness. There is also the other reference to the fact that he had only one-third of his whole available force mobilized in time for the battle. One further melancholy statement in the Worcester edition of the Chronicle adds a statement that Harold fought most resolutely against William but only 'with those men who wished to stand by him.' The writer was surely signalling much about Harold's unenviable plight here.

In taking a closer look at William's probable strength we must consider a number of balancing circumstances – how many men and horses his ships could have carried across the Channel, the losses he suffered at sea before he put into the haven of St Valery, losses by illness and accident and perhaps a few casualties due to ambushes by some gallant Anglo-Saxons in the peninsula, offset by additions in reinforcements from Normandy since 28 September and enrolment by some of the Norman residents in England and their retainers. Some of these factors are of course impossible to calculate accurately, but the most significant one – the capacity of his invasion fleet – does bear profitable examination. Modern investigators accept statements made at the time or shortly afterwards that William used about 700 ships to carry his forces across the Channel. The figure seems reasonable when we recall that Hardrada used 300 ships, most of them much bigger than William's to bring what he considered to be an adequate army to challenge Harold earlier in the autumn. Working on the tally of 700 ships and analysing clues and information offered in the Bayeux Tapestry and elsewhere, two well-equipped military specialists – Sir Charles Oman and Major-General E. R. James, of the Royal Engineers – came to strikingly similar verdicts about the size of William's army in studies made independently in 1907 and 1923. Others made this century have not been very far removed from these two assessments. Oman estimated the figure at between 11,000 and 12,000 altogether and General James at about 11,000.

This is not to say that William had all these men to put into battle. There had to be guards for the ships on the beach and the

equipment they had brought over from Normandy, garrisons for
the bases at Pevensey and Hastings, scouts posted round the
perimeter of the peninsula to give warning of any unexpected
English counter-assaults, and a large company of camp followers
for an assortment of non-combatant duties (including what must
have been a sizeable number of grooms and attendants for the
knights and the horses). We can reasonably put the number of all
these auxiliaries at about 3,000, and we therefore reach an approximate round figure of 8,000, or maybe a few more, as a rough
estimate of William's fighting strength. Lieutenant-Colonel
Lemmon, who lived for many years close to the battle area and
gave all the elements of the Hastings puzzle thorough attention,
goes further in his analysis of the composition of the fighting force
available to William. He divides a total of 8,000 into about 1,000
bowmen, 3,000 cavalry and 4,000 infantry. This calculation is
fundamentally conjectural, of course, but it is founded on a working lifetime as a professional soldier and is therefore entitled to
attention. Certainly, as one walks over and surveys the battlefield
of Hastings today, one can imagine the slopes below Senlac ridge
alive with anything up to 10,000 men and their horses, but not
more. Men and animals assembled in a company much greater than
that would, one feels, get unmanageably into each other's way.

In a consideration of Harold's probable fighting strength, different
factors are brought into play, and some of them work notably to
Harold's advantage. The core of his army was of course his Housecarls. These superb soldiers are thought to have numbered about
3,000 when at full strength, and this would seem to be about the
maximum number a Royal household could maintain as a permanent force close at hand. But there could not possibly have been
3,000 Housecarls with Harold at Senlac. Three weeks earlier this
elite corps of warriors had been through a fearful ordeal at Stamford Bridge, and although the Housecarls had won one of the finest
victories in the history of early English arms, they must have
suffered severely themselves. Most modern assessors agree that there
could not have been more than 2,000 Housecarls fit for action as
Harold's force assembled with him on 13 October on Caldbeck
Hill.

The rest of the army comprised mostly those thegns and their
personal detachments, plus the militiamen of the fyrd, who had
answered the summons to arms and had reached the Hoar Apple

Tree in time to be of use to the King; there were also the House-carls maintained by Harold's brothers, Gyrth and Leofwin. Their two earldoms comprised roughly East Anglia and Kent and were altogether much smaller than Harold's own former earldom of Wessex. They had no royal entitlement to volunteers from outside their own borders and consequently their corps of Housecarls would be much smaller than the King's. We may perhaps estimate these two subsidiary armies at a combined strength of some 2,000 men. Thus, adding them to Harold's available Housecarls, we get a figure of 4,000 for the basic professional force supporting him at Senlac. Would the thegnhood and the militia double that figure? Once more we have no hard information, but we do have some rough statistics upon which to build.

The population of England in the eleventh century has been confidently assessed at about a million and a half on the foundation of many figures extracted from the Domesday Survey. Domesday also indicates (according to some ingenious sums done by Professor Barlow in his biography of Edward the Confessor and other historians) that the rate of conscription for the whole of England just before the Conquest was about one soldier for every 70 to 100 inhabitants. This means that in theory the king could call up an army of between 15,000 and 20,000 men. But it would be unrealistic to infer that he would get anything like a full response to a call, even if he had the whole kingdom behind him. As Professor Barlow does, we shall be safe in estimating the maximum response to be about 10,000 men for both army and navy. But Harold could not count on anything like that kind of national reaction to his appeal, and in any case there was not time for all those who were willing to join him to arrive in time for the Battle of Hastings. A good guess might be that some 4,000 men joined the Housecarls at the Hoar Apple Tree, so that we eventually arrive at a total figure (albeit a conjectural one) of about 8,000 for Harold's gross mobilized strength.

In all the circumstances of time, national spirit or lack of it in many shires, the dimensions of Senlac ridge and the prolonged fighting to come on 14 October, it seems fairly safe to assume that there was no great disparity between the sizes of the opposing armies but that, since William was the attacker and had to suffer the greater losses during the long fight which he won, he must have been somewhat stronger.

An important point in all this estimating is that Harold was better placed than William in one respect. He could count on almost everybody around him being a fighting man so that although his total force of some 8,000 was considerably lower than William's, his percentage of effective fighting men was very much higher. He had no cavalry so that he did not have to detail men for service as grooms, attendants and the like. The Housecarls' ponies could be left loosely tethered close to the Andredsweald or committed to the care of local farmers and peasants, for their riders expected to be away in battle for only a short period, or for ever. Harold had also no need to allocate men to defend any rear bases or even to worry about attacks from any other source, for he had dealt decisively with foreign interference at Stamford Bridge and there was nobody else at home or abroad likely to assail him for quite a while. The lesson he had taught at Stamford Bridge must have been duly noted everywhere. Nor did he have to fear attrition by sickness, for any man who reached the Hoar Apple Tree would obviously be a fit man. Harold would be able to field at least 7,500 of the 8,000 men at his command on the eve of battle, and the figure would perhaps be slowly swelling as the hours passed and small groups of Englishmen turned up to join him.

So Harold had no doubt as to his ability to maintain by rota a day and night guard to pin down William inside the peninsula. The Senlac ridge from end to end was some 1,100 yards long. Allowing each warrior one yard of space to operate with his axe, bill, spear, or whatever other weapon he possessed, meant that there had to be only 1,100 men as front line defenders on the ridge at any one time. In case of emergency – and there was to be a supreme one less than 24 hours after the English had started gathering on Caldbeck Hill – Harold had enough men to form a shield-wall seven ranks deep, a formidable obstacle indeed to put against any attacker, especially one who had to come at the shield-wall up a slope.

Harold, to be sure, was in fair shape to make a good fight whatever happened. But not, as was soon to be tragically shown, a winning fight.

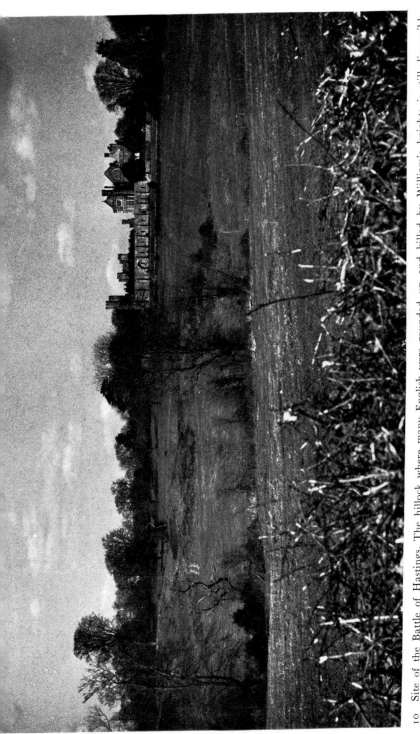

10 Site of the Battle of Hastings. The hillock where many English were rounded up and killed by William's knights is still discernible (left). Battle Abbey is in the background.

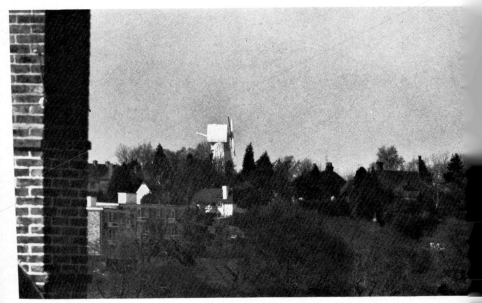

11 Caldbeck Windmill stands on the site of the Hoar Apple Tree where Harold assembled his troops for the battle.

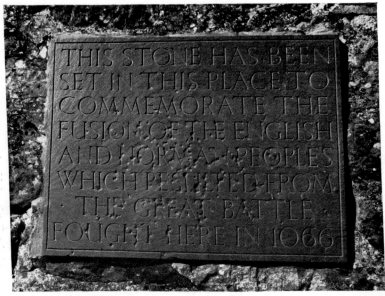

THIS STONE HAS BEEN
SET IN THIS PLACE TO
COMMEMORATE THE
FUSION OF THE ENGLISH
AND NORMAN PEOPLES
WHICH RESULTED FROM
THE GREAT BATTLE
FOUGHT HERE IN 1066

12 A stone set in 1966 to commemorate the Battle of Hastings was rapidly vandalised, presumably by anti-Norman dissenters.

9

The Battle

The air was moist, as ever in early morning in mid-October in England, but there was no rain when William's men began gathering for battle. Had the weather been at all unusual – if there had been rain, gale, fog or other visitation that day, the Tapestry and the chroniclers would surely have mentioned it, if only to glorify William's performance – the course of the battle would have been sharply changed, and in some circumstances decisively so. For example, if there had been a heavy autumnal storm coming in from the sea only seven miles away, the battle would probably not have been fought at all that day. One consequence of this would have been that Harold would have been granted the precious time he needed for his military salvation. He would have had a chance to receive laggard reinforcements, rest the most fatigued of his hard-driven troops and, above all, to have improved his defences by building a stout palisade and wide, deep ditch which, as we have noted, would have made his shield-wall virtually immune from Norman attack.

Thus a storm which enforced a postponement of battle could very well have ensured an English victory. There were other possible vagaries, not perhaps so potent in their scope but which would nevertheless have worked in favour of Harold. For example, anything heavier than a mere drizzle during Friday night would have made the soft Sussex turf too slippery for William's cavalry to canter or gallop up the slope to the ridge, or even to climb it at all. Rain would also have seriously interfered with the assault by hampering the movements of the archers and even affecting the efficiency of their bowstrings. It would also weigh down and tire heavily accoutred men-at-arms as they plodded uphill on soft and treacherous ground.

Speculation about the effects of weather is illuminating, for it emphasizes an important fundamental in military history. This is that the timing, course and outcome of many a battle – including some fought at sea by warships manoeuvring against each other in conditions far more volatile and mischievous than on land – have been dictated by weather. Some of the encounters which have shaped the fate of nations for generations would have developed very differently if the weather had been otherwise that day, or if it had caused a postponement of conflict. Hastings was one of these.

As it happened, the weather was again as kind to William on 14 October as it seems to have been, except initially, throughout his campaign. William's good fortune seems to have been due to an unusual pattern of weather in England and northern Europe during the eleventh century. Scientists who have pored over all the known records report that by the middle of the century one of the most benign periods of climate in documented English history had begun. There had been a period of severe cold for several centuries, but by 1066 the average temperature appears to have risen markedly. Summers were warm and sunny and winters relatively mild. The improvement had started only just in time to favour William, for the Anglo-Saxon Chronicle records that as late as 1047 'came the severe winter with frost and snow and widespread storms; it was so severe that no living man could remember another like it, because of the mortality of both men and cattle. Both birds and fish perished because of the hard frost and from hunger.' The change seems also to have been marked by a disturbance in the earth's crust in England, for on 1 May 1049, the rare phenomenon of an earthquake struck the midlands (at Worcester, Droitwich, Derby and elsewhere), killing many men and beasts and causing great damage by fire in Derbyshire. The benign period which apparently started immediately thereafter is estimated by climatologists to have lasted until about 1300.

Dawn broke at almost exactly 5.30 am on 14 October 1066, after a night dimly lit by a waning moon of less than half size. William's men must have been on the move very soon thereafter because, it is estimated, they had marched to the battlefield, seven miles north of Hastings, by about 9 am. They had not all been quartered in the tiny port of Hastings. Many of them had been dispersed in all the sheltered encampments they could find or make for themselves in the undulating, partly-wooded country of the Pevensey peninsula.

They must have made a sombre picture after they had assembled and started their trek to the battlefield. They would all converge from their billets upon the London–Hastings track, forming an eventual crocodile procession two to three miles long; thousands of them walking towards the Senlac meadow – archers and other infantrymen trudging along stolidly; high-born knights walking alongside their horses, across whose backs lay the chain mail the warriors would don later; small wooden carts with crudely-made wheels rasping and creaking as they rolled along with their burden of arms and stores; sergeants and other outriders rallying laggards and enforcing some kind of order in the procession. All the fighting men were there except those in the defensive screen of archers, men-at-arms and the small detachment of cavalry which William would surely have left overnight across the base of Senlac meadow as a precaution against any night-time raids from the ridge above. With the coming of daylight the few hundreds of Norman outposts must have been awaiting the coming of the main army with increasing anxiety. They must have felt naked and exposed as they warily watched for signs of any offensive movement in the English line ranged menacingly against them a few hundred yards away at the top of the meadow.

William had planned everything carefully, as usual. With his personal bodyguard and probably one or two of his closest friends and sub-commanders, he rode on ahead of his army soon after dawn to an intermediate command post which he had chosen in advance as his equivalent of the Hoar Apple Tree. It has been identified with some certainty as Blackhorse Hill (440 feet), the highest point on Telham Hill and well over one mile short of the base of Senlac meadow. Blackhorse Hill stood conveniently alongside the London–Hastings track and was therefore highly suitable as a spot where William could show himself prominently and inspire his men with a display of confidence and high spirit as he directed them forward to their allotted places in Senlac meadow.

As he carried out this commander's duty he was comparatively close to Harold, perhaps a mile and a half away assuming that Harold was similarly occupied behind the ridge, but they could not see each other's position because of the rises and falls in the country which separated them. The English battle line only came into view about half a mile further on from Blackhorse Hill, at a point on the London–Hastings track where this ran through what are now the grounds of Telham Court. It must have been from this locality, or somewhere close to it, that Norman scouts kept watch on the English lines and rode back in relays to Blackhorse Hill to report any activity to William, as he sat there in full armour at his command post. They would give him an estimate of the size of the English force, how it was being disposed along the ridge and what preparatory moves the English were making for the action so close at hand. And, as the Bayeux Tapestry graphically and artistic- ally depicts, Harold's scouts were waiting and watching behind clumps of trees near Senlac to observe the Norman approach and send back similar reports to Harold.

William of Poitiers by no means misses the opportunity to use his imagination in describing this phase of the advance to the battle area. He relates pompously that 'with great humility' Duke William had hung round his neck the relics upon which, he claimed, Harold had sworn an oath which he had since renounced. With ludicrous naïvety, the scribe then states that, although nobody had reported to him in detail the short harangue which he says William gave his troops on Blackhorse Hill, 'we doubt not that it was excellent.' The Norman propagandist traps himself here, for he asks us to believe that the Duke gave an 'excellent' address to several thousand men straggling along about two miles of winding track. He then strains trust beyond all charitable limits by quoting the very words which he has just disclosed nobody had relayed to him.

The imagined recital was a mish-mash of lofty exhortation and terrible warning of what would happen to the soldiers if the battle were lost. 'You fight', the scribe reports William as saying, 'not merely for victory but also for survival. If you bear yourselves valiantly you will obtain victory, honour and riches. If not, you will be ruthlessly butchered, or else led ignominiously captive into the hands of pitiless enemies. Further, you will incur abiding dis- grace. There is no road for retreat. In front, your advance is blocked by an army and a hostile countryside; behind you, there is the sea where the enemy fleet bars your flight. The English have again and again fallen to the sword of an enemy; often, being vanquished, they have submitted to a foreign yoke; nor have they ever been famed as soldiers. The vigorous courage of a few men armed in a just cause and specially protected from Heaven must prevail against a host of men unskilled in combat. Only be bold so that nothing shall make you yield, and victory will gladden your hearts.'*

This piece of prose is of intense interest even though it is mostly fictional and heightens mistrust in William of Poitiers as a strictly factual reporter. He was writing as Duke William's semi-official mouthpiece and his version of his master's words must therefore be interpreted as, in its essentials, reflecting the Duke's assessment of the Norman situation and the frame of mind in which he led his men into battle. The passage does expose some of the fundamental elements of William's spectacular enterprise and is of great help in analysing this phase of the Conquest. He never spoke the actual words attributed to him but they must be accepted as conveying what was in his mind as his men filed past him on Blackhorse Hill. He knew that for them, as for him, everything was at stake this day.

The horses and store wagons and the rest of the paraphernalia needed to sustain the attack, are estimated to have passed William by 8 am. He now rode through them to the place on the battlefield itself from which he directed their precise deployment for action. This was a spot, still identifiable, at which the track to London began its ascent from the bottom of Senlac meadow towards the ridge straddled by Harold's army. The deployment was ordered by William from a knoll (now cut through by a railway) and he operated in full view of Harold, who was now little more than 200 yards distant up the modest slope.

Harold apparently did nothing whatever to harass the Normans while they were forming up for action against him. Some observers have suggested that this passivity was in accord with some rough tradition of the era by which nobody attacked until the battle had formally opened, with ruffles and flourishes as it were. Maybe so, but a much stronger and more likely reason is available in these particular circumstances. Harold knew that to send his House-carls and fyrdmen tearing down the hill to hurl themselves upon the Normans before they were ready for battle would have gained only a fleeting advantage and would have led to his sure defeat. His men would have been able to cause initial havoc and slaughter, but once the Normans rallied from the surprise, their cavalry would assuredly cut the English to pieces; there would be no

* David C. Douglas and George W. Greenaway, *English Historical Documents* (Eyre and Spottiswoode, 1968).

withstanding their speed, mobility and sheer weapon-power as they wheeled and plunged against the Saxon infantrymen from their superior stance on horseback.

The plain truth is that Harold had only one clear hope for victory, and his tactic in massing his forces tightly along Senlac ridge shows that he knew this and planned to act accordingly. He intended to hold his men doggedly on the defensive behind their shield-wall, on higher ground than the assaulting enemy. Military history in England and northern Europe offered him evidence in plenty that skilled and determined defenders could withstand attack almost indefinitely provided they were not overwhelmingly out-numbered but were ensconced in an advantageous position, were firmly led and did not suffer some totally unexpected disaster during combat. Further, Harold could calculate with some justi-fication that William's losses as the attacker would be greater than his own and that consequently there should come a moment of opportunity for him. Since he could now plainly see that while William was numerically the stronger he was not overwhelmingly so, there was a good chance that before the day was done the Norman infantry and cavalry would become so thinned out that it would be safe for the English, even without cavalry, to burst at last from their position on the ridge and pursue the remnants of William's force back to the sea or destroy them as they fled there. Such, at any rate, must have been his hope.

Senlac ridge was suitable to the kind of resolute, if nerve-racking and frustrating, defence which Harold planned. Besides providing the comparatively short front of 1,100 yards which he could protect in formidable depth, it could not be side-tracked by Normans sneaking round it to the right or the left because these flanks were sealed by rapidly falling ground split up by ravines. Some of these were very deep, carrying streams and trailing off eventually into marshy ground unsuitable for use by either cavalry or infantry. This sealing off was one of the natural attributes which made the northerly bottleneck of the Pevensey peninsula such an attractive front for Harold. His army was in effect perched on high, dry ground to which it had easy access from the Hoar Apple Tree by a narrow saddle of land carrying the London-Hastings track. The highest point of the ridge (275 feet) was a hillock slightly to east of centre of the ridge, and it was here that Harold naturally took his commander's position with his two battle flags – believed to have been The Dragon of Wessex and Harold's personal standard, The Fighting Man – planted on either side of him.

From this dominating position he watched William's men stream across the bottom of the meadow and form up into three blocks approximately 175 feet lower than the ridge. The open meadow sloped gently down from the gorse-covered ridge. The gradients are estimated to have been 1 in 15 from the place where Harold stood, 1 in 35 at the western end of the shield-wall, and 1 in 22 to the east. (These mild descents compare with gradients of between 1 in 4 and 1 in 6 which the painstaking Colonel Lemmon says guarded Harold's flanks to the rear.)

William's three divisions were alike in composition. Each comprised a front rank of archers, a second of men-at-arms and a third of cavalry. The centre division, the core of the army and technically under the personal command of William, was probably about twice the size of each of the other two. The one on the right flank was made up of French and Flemish troops and was under the command of Roger de Montgomerie. Roger's family originated in Calvados, the same area from which Wiliam's hailed, and since they had presumably grown up together it was entirely appropriate that William should have had as, literally, his right hand man in battle the comrade of his boyhood. Roger's division faced the curving left flank of Harold's army and, like it, straddled the London-Hastings track.

The men in William's centre bloc, which was perhaps 3,000 strong, were his elite troops. They were mostly his fellow-Normans and they were the equivalent of Harold's Housecarls, men who were always closest to him in battle and whom he knew he could trust to fight for him devotedly, if necessary to the death. Although William now raised his standard and his papal banner in their midst to indicate his presence with them, he obviously had far wider preoccupations this day than the usual personal command of them. He had arranged to delegate field-control of this central bloc of choice troops and knights to his two half-brothers. One was Odo, the fighting bishop; the other Robert, Count of Mortain. Robert had an advantage over his two half-brothers, for he did not share their stigma of illegitimacy, having been borne in all marital propriety by Arletta, their mother, after she had married and become the Countess de Conteville.

(Robert was to be handsomely rewarded for his share in the

victory at Senlac, for in the first share-out of the spoils thereafter, William gave him lands in Sussex, and advanced him later by appointing him Duke of Cornwall. He was faithful unto William's death. He was one of the few who stood at the Conqueror's bed-side when he died in miserably squalid circumstances soon after dawn on 9 September 1087, at Nantes, on the estuary of the river Loire. William had had to dash back to Normandy from England to drive out invaders from his Duchy. He was by this time old and overweight, but he was still an accomplished commander and he scored one final brilliant victory over his challengers. He emphasized it by burning and sacking the town of Nantes – but as he rode away through the smoking ruins his horse stumbled over a still lively ember and William was pitched forward so violently that he collapsed to the ground with his intestines badly ruptured. He lin-gered in intermittent agony for 12 days before he died.)

William's third division lay to his left on low, flat ground close to what is now the playing field of Battle Abbey School. This bloc was composed of Bretons and men from Maine and Anjou and was commanded by Alan Fergent, Count of Brittany. These troops were deployed on the lowest corner of the battlefield, slightly less than 200 feet above sea level, and they and their horses stood not on firm turf but on spongy marshland which degenerated behind them into swamps. Ahead of them the ground rose gently but steadily towards Senlac ridge and once they advanced the going would soon become firm and good.

Opposing this neatly-marshalled and, as it would seem from the orderly massing which they carried out, well-trained army were the English standing to their arms in a thick and slightly curving line at the top of the meadow. They were mostly facing south-east with the strengthening October light against their faces. (One chronicler mentions that when William and his knights were ad-vancing towards Senlac they carried some of their armour instead of wearing it because the day was already so warm; nobody has left any word about whether the sun shone on 14 October 1066, so perhaps it was one of those typical English 'nice days' when the sun tries valiantly to pierce through the cloud cover but never quite manages to do so.) The English were arrayed and armed to fight the kind of battle to which they and their Viking and Anglo-Saxon ancestors had been used for so long – the primitive, bestial clash in which men stood in opposing lines with just enough room between each man for the sword and the axe to be whirled and thrust until, at last, one side began to falter and the demoralized survivors of the appalling slaughter to which it had been exposed turned round and fled the field. Such a clash was always grimly decisive. The beaten side would never reassemble and take the field again for another fight because whatever cohesive spirit it had had was dissipated by the physical dismemberment (in more than one sense) suffered in its defeat. The winners would usually be so exhausted and mauled themselves that they could neither give chase that same day nor, for many another day, regroup to fight again as an army.

William's Plan

But today's encounter was to be a very different kind of affair. It was to inaugurate or at least confirm a new concept of warfare – one of co-ordination of different forms of mobile attack against a stationary enemy – which was to continue to be developed in ever-broadening scope until the twentieth century, when the coming of fearsome nuclear power of obliteration changed everything. Nobody can know today exactly what happened on that hill outside Hastings in 1066. But if we discard the blatantly flowery and biassed passages written into the Anglo-Norman versions of the event produced by scribes as long as a century afterwards, we can get somewhere. In particular we can accept such believable and confirmed evidence as exists, and use the careful analyses produced after years of research, both at Senlac and in the archives, by military experts such as Sir Charles Oman, Lieutenant-Colonel Burne, Lieutenant-Colonel Lemmon and Brigadier C. N. Barclay. In ignoring all other material, we shall be missing much of the exciting individual action, for of course not everything written by the post-Conquest poets and chroniclers was false or invented. But we shall still have a story thrilling enough if we keep within the bounds of known fact and likely probability.

William's battle plan is clear from the composition of his divisions and the way he arrayed them in three separate units which would attack as independent sub-armies but in co-ordination. The bowmen would be the first to strike by marching forward ahead of their comrades on foot and on horseback. Once within range they would shower the English with relays of arrows. They would then retire and the men-at-arms would march through them to tackle the harassed enemy at close quarters. When they too were spent, they would fall back to make way for the mounted knights to plunge through any gaps which had been made in the enemy line and, wheeling round, cut down as many victims as they could before they also retired to regroup. The men-at-arms and the knights would assuredly leave behind some, perhaps many, of their number as casualties but this was warfare of the particularly bloody kind practised in medieval times and a high proportion of casualties was inevitable and accepted. William estimated, or at least had to hope, that he would have enough men and mounts to repeat the procedure again and again until the thinned and tormented English lost heart and turned and ran.

William's strategy was revolutionary. Archers, infantry and cavalry had been used before in continental warfare, of course, but probably never before had a commander planned to use them to-gether with such precision – in sharp rotation to secure maximum cumulative effect from their specialized blows. His decision to divide his army into three homogeneous entities also reflected his imaginative thinking. Men in each of his three blocs were, as completely as could be arranged, natives of a particular region so that they had the advantage and comfort of close communal feeling. (In the same way, in later centuries, the English and European county and provincial regiments, and American state divisions, had a core of men whose families had lived close together for generations.) The sub-dividing of William's army brought him another benefit. If one division failed to dent the English shield-wall, one of the other two might succeed in so doing; in other words he had three chances of success instead of one. We can be sure that during the weeks of enforced waiting for the right wind William had drilled his men regularly and thoroughly so that they knew what was expected of them when they went into action and would carry out their manoeuvres quickly and without confusion. He had probably hoped that he would not have to ask them to attack uphill and on such a narrow front, offering no chance of taking their enemy on the flank, but there was nothing he could do to alter that.

One thing William did not know was the influence which his

tactics at Hastings were to have upon military history. His archers were the forerunners of the modern artillerymen. They fired off their missiles by hand whereas the later gunners would operate away to the rear and indirectly, via complicated devices and machinery; but the purpose was the same – to 'soften up' the enemy, in the horrible euphemism for killing and maiming, as a preliminary to shock attack. His knights were the predecessors of the men in armoured cars and tanks who would punch their way through the enemy ranks in such famous battles as those in which the Americans sent Germans recoiling out of France in 1945 and the British and their Commonwealth allies finally routed Rommel and his Afrika Korps in the Western Desert of Africa at El Alamein in 1942.

Battle Joined

The battle started fairly late in the morning. Some moment between 9 and 10 am is a good estimate in view of the four or five hours it must have taken the Norman detachments to reach Senlac and form up in their prescribed lines and positions. One imagines William giving the signal to start the attack only after riding up and down the lines of his three divisions to make sure that not only his sub-commanders but all their men knew exactly what he expected of them. This would surely have been the time for William to have made the 'excellent harangue' to his men mentioned by the versatile William of Poitiers as having been delivered on Telham Hill, for this was the moment when his men were keyed to the highest pitch of nervous expectation and needed all the encouragement they could get.

The first move came when the three thin lines of archers started marching forward up the slope of the meadow. They held their short, simply-made bows at the ready and their quivers full of arrows hung at their right hip from a stout belt slung around the waist; they would be silent and intent, their gaze fixed upon the target coming closer into range with every step. Trumpets had sounded to tell the archers to move off and the thin notes were borne upon the air towards the English shield-wall on the ridge, stirring hearts into faster rhythm and tensing the muscles of faces toughened by years of exposure to sun, wind and rain. Men would take a tighter, more comforting grip of their weapons. Some would exchange grim and not very funny jokes, to mask the fear. Surely, men would tell each other the Old English equivalent of 'Get ready to duck, mate,' as their descendants did at corresponding moments in the First and Second World Wars, and doubtless in many other wars as well.

Although the English were by no means as physically rested as their enemies, who had not had to endure any fighting or exacting forced marches since they landed at Pevensey two weeks earlier, they were in good condition to withstand the first and probably the fiercest of the attacks upon them. The question was whether the demands which Harold had had to make upon so many of them since Hardrada had appeared in the north-east had sapped their staying power for a fierce battle which would almost certainly last until darkness fell. But they had had some 20 hours in which to put up impromptu defences along the ridge and get some rest before the battle. The front rank of the English was composed of veteran Housecarls and well-equipped thegns stationed at intervals between the poorer-armed and less experienced shire levies of the fyrd. All stood immediately behind shields shaped like kites. Warriors armed with bills and axes, which needed the use of two hands, had stuck the pointed bottoms of their shields into the turf. Others equipped with the short iron sword of the period had their shields hanging from the neck by a loose leather strap. They held the shield closely to their bodies by a leather loop through which they placed their left forearm. Behind these front-line soldiers was a mixed bag of six or seven supporting ranks of warriors of varying worth. There were men with spears and javelins; men with slings, studded maces, home-made swords and daggers, and there were also probably piles of reserve shovels, forks and other farm tools for use if the worst happened and some Normans did break through the shield-wall and come within striking distance of the last resisters of all.

The best troops in the front ranks of Harold's army, now bracing themselves for the first and fiercest shocks of combat, were naturally the best protected. They wore the same iron helmets with short oblong forepiece covering the nose as did the Normans, as well as the same kind of hauberk or mail shirt – a one-piece garment reaching from neck to knee and slitted at each side from the waist down so that the wearer could ride as well as walk at need. The less professional elements of the army were covered with whatever leather protective garb they could make for themselves or find somewhere, and a number of them carried rounded convex shields of limewood.

All stood there watching the sinister lines of archers moving unevenly, like an almost spent wave seeping in upon the sand of the shore, closer and closer. The English could see the men-at-arms carrying lances, swords and maces, forming up behind the archers. And behind them were William's knights. They had mounted their sweating and excited horses and were getting ready to follow the two forward detachments and ride through them as they fell back after they had done their duty – killing or maiming as many of the English as they could and inevitably leaving behind some fallen comrades of their own, destined to be ridden over by the knights as they swept up to the English line.

The archers paused when they came to within about 100 yards of the ridge. They were now within range of their target and out of range of any missiles which the English had ready to hurl towards them. Prudence demanded that these men – standing several feet apart to the left, the centre and the right of the English line – should not venture too close to their enemy, for most of them wore no defensive armour or even protective clothing of any kind. Archers had one of the most specialized but least dangerous missions of all the warriors in the medieval army, and they were particularly safe at Senlac today because the English had no archers of their own to fire retaliatory volleys at their tormentors. Even if they had, the Norman bowmen would be fairly safe since they were spaced widely apart across the meadow and thus each made a hard mark to hit.

They now fired their first volley. They did not kneel to take aim and loose their shafts. They stood with their legs widely separated fore and aft, almost like runners set to start a race, and with a practised professionalism took a quick aim at the shield-wall and fired away their stout wooden arrows capped with deadly sharp metal points. Seeing the shower of missiles flying towards them, the English crouched behind their shields and whatever other protection they had managed to secure. One volley was followed by another but most of the arrows did little harm since the English were fresh and alert. As the Tapestry clearly depicts, most of the

arrows were safely fielded, but some at least must have found a
mark to draw first blood on what was to prove a day of frightful
slaughter. There is no record of how many volleys the archers let
loose on this first assault but, for what it is worth as a pointer, the
Tapestry shows the Norman archers to be carrying up to half a
dozen arrows in their quivers; the likelihood is that this was merely
an indication and that the bowmen in fact carried many more than
six. Whatever the number, the opening attack could not have been
very prolonged because there was only a one-way traffic in arrows.
Harold may have had just a few archers, but there could have
been no significant flow of spent English arrows for the Normans
to pick up and send back. In effect, once an archer had fired
off his own supply, he was out of action until fresh arrows were
brought to him from the rear or he had retired to pick them up
for himself.

Amid presumably some groans and screams from the few English
who had been hit and amid angry shouts and taunts from the mass
of relieved survivors after the opening barrage, the archers made
way for the men-at-arms to pass through their line up the hill. Their
work was temporarily accomplished, for once the men-at-arms
came within 10 or 15 yards of the shield-wall, friendly arrows
would have picked them off even more easily than they would the
English behind the protection of their shields

Now came the first hand-to-hand combat of the day. Those of the
Norman infantry who had not been felled by the fusillade of lances
and javelins, or had their skulls cracked open or their bones broken
by jagged, heavy stones tightly tied to wooden handles (the forerunners of the hand grenade) hurled at them as they made the last
few yards towards the shield-wall, fared none too rosily at the hands
of the stalwart Housecarls and the fresh and spirited fyrdmen
wielding bills, battle axes and swords. The Norman chroniclers all
bear witness to the toughness of the English during this early
phase of the battle, and with good reason. The men-at-arms were
undoubtedly sent back reeling without having made dents of any
consequence in the English line for exploitation by the knights,
who came galloping up the ridge. Presumably, one or two knights
were able to force a way through small gaps in the front line of
the defenders and made some bloody havoc with their whirling
swords and jabbing lances, but these over-daring members of
William's elite could not have survived. Horses as well as riders

would be quickly brought down and unhorsed knights would be hacked to pieces by the mass of the English surrounding them so thickly.

A Drawn Round

William's first combined attack by his archers, infantrymen and cavalry, failed disastrously and almost conclusively. The clang and clatter of the battle, offset by a hideous refrain of screams from men in agony, squeals of fear and pain from injured horses, and shouts and curses from men all but demented by the awful ecstasy of combat, ended abruptly. The morale of the Breton division on William's left wing suddenly broke. This division had been the first to come to close grips with the English because it had had the gentlest slope of all (1 in 33) to tackle. But it had plunged headlong into much more spirited defence than it had expected, and it quickly found itself fighting against heavy odds with its right flank unsupported because the Normans in the centre had taken much longer to finish their more exacting climb of 1 in 15 and had then also found themselves stopped short by the fury of the English defence as they surged towards the shield-wall.

The Bretons broke off fighting and turned away. Alan Fergent's knights, temporarily bewildered and unnerved, galloped off down-hill to retrieve their composure and prepare themselves for the next assault which they knew the unrelenting William would demand of them. They were followed by a disordered rabble of unhorsed riders, infantrymen and archers stumbling back towards their swampy base at the bottom left of the meadow. It looked like a humiliating and decisive rout. The sight of their enemy staggering away thus was too much for the excited English at the western end of the shield-wall. Recklessly, forgetting all caution, they burst forth from behind their shields and tore off downhill after the fleeing Bretons. Seeing this ominous debacle developing on their left flank, the men of William's two other divisions wavered. There was the possibility that the rest of the English would follow the example of those of their comrades who had broken out to give chase and would come at the central division from its unprotected flank. This division thereupon broke off its attack and prudently fell back but in much more orderly style than the Bretons. Momentarily, it looked possible that the battle was over before it had properly started and that the English had a stunning victory within their grasp. This would probably have been so against a less resolute and slower-thinking field general than William.

He responded instantly to the threatening challenge. He galloped forward from his command post at the bottom centre of Senlac meadow, blocked the retreat of the Normans under Odo and Robert of Mortain and in so doing curbed a similar incipient movement among the French and Flemings under Roger de Montgomerie on his right. It was too late for him to do anything to restore quickly the cohesion of the routed and dispersed Bretons. But he had perceived a way of exacting a merciless profit from the foolishness of those headstrong English who had put themselves within his power by abandoning the sanctuary of their shield-wall. He ordered knights from his still-effective Norman division to wheel westwards across the field and cut down the pursuing fyrdmen, now hopelessly cut off from any help from Harold. They were driven towards and rounded up on a hillock (which is still believed to be identifiable less than 100 yards uphill from a fishpond occupying some of the swampy land of 1066). Again, the Tapestry catches a moment of drama in the battle; it shows the headstrong English being despatched by William's horsemen surrounding the hillock. There could not have been more than a handful of survivors from this tragic episode. Only the last of those men who had abandoned the shield-wall and had not yet had time to run as far downhill as the hillock would have any chance of turning round and regaining the ridge.

One can imagine the horror and anger with which Harold watched the massacre from his command post on the highest part of the ridge. Looking over the heads of the men ranged around and in front of him Harold would see it all only too clearly. Impotent to help because by doing so he would only compound the disaster, he could but make sure that the depleted line to his right was reformed and restored in time to meet the next assault, which would not be long in coming now that William had not only staved off disaster but had profited from it. The fatal rashness of the inexperienced levies had depressingly confirmed the correctness of Harold's conviction that victory, even survival, depended upon his men standing firm behind the shield-wall, against no matter what temptation or provocation, until William's forces had been broken up and were no longer capable of attack.

There was now a pause, badly needed by both sides. Each commander had to repair damage and digest the lessons of the first violent clash. It had really ended in a draw. William's assault had failed because it had not pierced the shield-wall and but for his quick thinking might have ended in his utter defeat. As for Harold, his line had held magnificently, but this encouraging early success had been badly marred by the foolish indiscipline of his fyrdmen.

William's prime concern was with his Bretons, whose inexperience had let him down so dangerously. These were the 'greenest' troops of all in William's army, many of them never having been in action before. They had been recruited from primitive rural areas and were a remarkably diverse company. It has been established* that among them were former bandits who were notorious because they painted their faces black to avoid being recognized while following their profession; from them comes the surname of Talbot from the Old French word *talebot*, meaning lamp black. These were among the men who, perhaps understandably, recoiled when their presumed victims in the shield-wall showed infinitely more fight than they had expected. We can see William cantering over to the lower left of Senlac field to admonish the shamefaced Bretons as they slowly recovered their composure. Next time they must be steadier, must keep an eye upon the men in his own division on their right and advance in step with them, and even if they found once again that the blows dealt them by the English at close quarters were so fierce as to blunt their attack without a breakthrough, they must retire in good order, again in step with the centre division, and not in panic. They must realize that every attack they made would assuredly thin the human fabric of the shield-wall, and sooner or later the English must weaken against the co-ordinated onslaughts being made against them.

As for Harold, his one vital task was to make sure that his fyrdmen did not repeat their rashness. They would not need much convincing, for they had seen what William's cavalrymen had done to those who had given in to the temptations of pursuit.

There were other tasks for the English during this lull, most of them unpleasant. Dead and wounded defenders had to be passed

* By H. Moisy, in his *Noms de famille Normands*, (Paris, 1875).

to the rear, to receive the meagre and primitive ministrations of non-combatant camp followers, perhaps even one or two women who were the forerunners of the nurses of later centuries of warfare. Gaps in the front ranks of the shield-wall had to be filled and the whole line had to be straightened and, wherever possible, strengthened at points which had shown weakness against the onset of the Normans. The corpses of dead enemy infantrymen, knights and horses must be hauled out in front of the shield-wall to become grisly obstacles in the path of the next waves of attackers. We do not know for sure what happened to those enemy wounded who could not stumble or crawl off down the slope to safety among their comrades, but we can guess. They would be shown little pity beyond a quick despatch. The age of chivalry had not yet dawned.

It must have been close to midday when William started his next assault up the hill. Again the archers, their quivers refilled, advanced to let loose their debilitating barrage. Again the men-at-arms strode through the line of bowmen – who kept on firing their volleys while the infantrymen were plodding on ahead of them – to fight their crude and bloody duel with the Housecarls and the fyrdmen; and again thereafter the Norman knights rode upon the bristling English line on the ridge. This time there was no Norman debacle. But neither was the shield-wall decisively breached; there were plenty of the English still on their feet.

William must have had some evidence, however, to confirm to him that his tactics were succeeding, for he persevered with them again and again, following up the barrages of flying missiles with bodily assaults by infantry and horsemen. His losses mounted with every attack, but so did those of the English and Harold had unnerving evidence, probably during the early afternoon, that the Norman knights were at last managing to pierce the thinning English line. Two of his brothers, Gyrth and Leofwin, were killed one after the other. Their fall tells a story of Norman incursion deep into the English ranks, for Gyrth and Leofwin were among Harold's principal lieutenants and they would not be fighting in the front ranks of the defenders but, like Harold, from commanding positions towards the rear. Normans must have been penetrating deep to be able to cut them down.

Even William had a close call. As the fighting became fiercer and his men needed all the encouragement they could get to face yet again the murderous blows the English were dealing them,

William joined them in their advance up the hill. Never a commander to shrink personal exposure to danger, he rode to the
shield-wall with the knights of his Norman division and laid about
him with his sword. Suddenly he was seen to go down off his horse
and the word spread quickly among his men that he had been
killed. What had happened was that his mount had been cut down
by some Housecarl. His men closed round him as he lay prostrate
to protect him from further harm while another horse was quickly
found for him. He re-mounted and, as one panel of the Tapestry
illustrates, he lifted the visor of his helmet so that those near him
should recognize him and spread the news that he was alive and
unhurt. The Tapestry shows Eustace of Boulogne (the same man
who 16 years earlier had provoked the discreditable scuffle at Dover
which contributed to the banishment of Harold and the rest of the
Godwin family) pointing to William to draw attention to the proof
he is giving of his survival.

Inevitably, both sides began to flag as the afternoon wore on.
The English must have been still fighting dourly, for there is no
evidence anywhere that the Normans were overwhelming them,
even though the attackers were apparently making intermittent
breaches in the shield-wall as the ranks of the defenders were
steadily depleted and their line inevitably shortened. Harold's one
hope now was that his men would be able to hold out until night-
fall, a few minutes after six o'clock; his other hope that William's
casualties would become too numerous to bear was not being fulfilled. The weight and mobility of cavalry was working for William
as he had calculated. If he had had only bowmen and infantry it
would have been perfectly feasible, and likely, that Harold would
have staged a mass charge downhill and swept them off the field.
But, as had been proved by the early disaster which befell the
surging levies – a disaster which, if the Norman chroniclers are to
be believed, was repeated during the afternoon when William
ordered a feigned flight of his men – the menace of the cavalry
operating alternately with the bowmen dictated immobility upon
Harold. The passive defence which he was being forced to make
was entirely out of keeping with both his character and soldierly
training, and it is a tribute to his strength of mind that he apparently
followed it to the end.

Harold Falls

This came to him, it is surmised, just after 5 pm. It was caused by yet another stratagem which the wily William contrived as he strove to gain the victory which he must have before darkness frustrated him and gave his stubborn enemy a night in which to receive more reinforcements and face him refreshed on the morrow. William's inspiration was to tell his archers to change their angle of fire – to lift their bows in front so that their arrows would clear the brandished shields of the first line of English and fall down upon the middle and rear ranks of soldiers who would not be expecting them in such a shower.

The ruse may have occurred to William because in the confused state of the fighting late in the day he was not able to use his archers as effectively as earlier on, for it is inconceivable that the battle should have remained formalized, in the manner in which it started, for six or seven hours. His infantrymen and knights could not have kept their precise formations for so long throughout so many advances and retreats. Men from one division would merge with those of another as a small group of attackers on foot or mounted managed to make a temporary breach in the shield-wall and others hurried to join them in exploiting it. The result of such *mêlées* would be that it would become unsafe for the archers to fire as they had been doing, for fear of hitting their own comrades engaged almost hand-to-hand with the enemy.

Whatever the explanation, the Tapestry shows William's archers obeying his new order. In the lower border of a panel illustrating an unequal combat between a galloping knight and an English Housecarl, the archers are seen with their bows tilted upwards and their gaze uplifted; they are obviously taking aim at a much higher angle than is shown in the earlier pictures of them in action.

The ruse brought William decisive dividends. Men fighting around Harold at his command post towards the rear of the English lines were wounded and killed by arrows coming so unexpectedly upon them from aloft. A legend has persisted that Harold was himself fatally wounded in the right eye by one of the arrows. This seems not to be true. It was started over 30 years after the battle by Baudri, Abbot of Bourgeuil, in a poem in which he infers that a contemporary tapestry, almost certainly the Bayeux Tapestry, depicts the episode. This is not so. The warrior seen falling with an arrow in the eye is one of the men close to Harold, a sub-commander or one of his advisers, and Baudri was led into misreading the Tapestry because the wording, 'Hic Harold Rex Interfectus Est' (Here King Harold is killed) straddles two panels, but in the judgement of almost every expert who has examined the Tapestry it refers to the second panel. In this Harold is seen being cut down by the sword of a Norman knight.

What appears to have happened in this final, climactic phase of the battle is that the volleys of the Norman archers did in fact win the day for William without fatally wounding Harold. They caused casualties not only close to him but all along the rearward ranks of the thinned shield-wall, and this fresh setback so weakened the morale of the English fighting for their lives in the fading October light that the line at last gave way. A party of some twenty knights was able to hack a path through it towards Harold's position just off the London-Hastings track, and four of the knights survived to reach him. One chronicler (William of Malmesbury) names them as: Ivo de Ponthieu, Clifford the Younger, Mountfort, and the ubiquitous Eustace of Boulogne. They struck at Harold with their swords, wounding him fearfully, and one of them, said to be Ivo, went on cutting off his limbs after he was dead. For this piece of unnecessary and unworthy savagery he was, again according to William of Malmesbury, expelled from the Norman army and sent home in disgrace.

Harold's fall brought William's victory. As news of the King's death spread through the remnants of his army, and was harshly confirmed by the inrush of more and more knights through gaping spaces in the dissolving shield-wall, English resistance collapsed at last. A few groups of warriors stood firm here and there to fight to the end, but most of the English are believed to have fled the field soon after Harold's death and made for the Andredsweald, whose dense forestry gave obscurity and shelter. Although the English appear to have fought so stubbornly as a whole on this awful day, some suspicion arises that desertions might have been occurring during the afternoon as some of the fyrdmen perceived that the Norman attacks were not lessening in ferocity and the ordeal of meeting them was becoming more and more exacting and dangerous. One ponders again that loaded entry in the Chronicle: 'Nevertheless, the King fought against him (William) most resolutely with those men who wished to stand with him.' The

English monk was undoubtedly indicating the shortcoming in the response to Harold's call to arms before the battle. But was he also trying to suggest desertions during the battle?

Dusk was at hand by the time William's tired but triumphant troops had stilled all resistance to them, for there is no acceptable evidence of anything but token pursuit of their fleeing enemies in the aftermath of battle. The minor effort which appears to have been made on orders of William but with some reluctance by Eustace of Boulogne, the man commanded by William to organize it, ended suddenly. Knights sent by Eustace to ride in the fading light towards the Andredsweald tumbled one after another into a wide and deep ditch which later became known with justification as Malfosse but has never been satisfactorily located. Even if this disaster had not checked the hunters after the English, they would not have been able to give chase for very much longer. Pursuit by night was impossible because there was to be no moon until midnight and it would then be only a small one and would keep low in the skies. Modern horsemen who have experimented near the battlefield have found that even in good conditions in mid-October it was hazardous to ride anywhere around the Senlac meadow at 6 pm and was out of the question a quarter of an hour later.

So we may safely assume that William allowed his knights to rest soon after the fight had been won, leaving these weary English remnants to straggle off into the night as best they could. It is said that William then ordered one part of the battlefield to be cleared of its shocking debris so that some kind of a tent could be put up. He ordered champagne to be brought to him – not the bubbling kind we know today but still white wine from vineyards established in Champagne by the Romans. (The device of keeping sparkle in wine by means of a cork in a bottle was not discovered until after 1600 by an enterprising monk at Hautvillers.)

Looters, and perhaps a few grieving English searching for the remains of their fallen menfolk, began roaming the field next day. What happened to the most renowned, and perhaps the most tragic, victim of them all – Harold, last of the Saxon Kings – is not known. One romantic story which has been handed down to us is that Edith Swan Neck had to be summoned to identify his mangled body and that she did so by verifying marks upon it known to her as his mistress. One clerk recording the history of Waltham Abbey describes Edith Swan Neck as 'a clever woman'. Recounting the story of her identification of the body of Harold after the battle, he says, 'she seemed more fitted than any others to determine this matter, who recognized him whom she sought among thousands of the dead, the more easily because she had lovingly looked after the clothes of him whom she loved and greatly influenced, inasmuch as she was known to have been freely admitted to the secrets of his bed.' Another of the unidentified scribes puts the same thing in different words. He writes that Edith was 'a woman whom he had known before he assumed the kingship of the English. She shared the lord King's bedchamber wherever he went and knew better than others secret marks on him, being admitted to his inmost secrets.'

It has also been said that William, vindictively, would not let her or Harold's mother take the body away for ceremonial burial. Perhaps he did not wish any form of shrine to be created and used as a rallying place for the opposition and even the hatred that he knew the English would feel towards him – an alien aggressor and conqueror. One tale has it that he contemptuously ordered Harold to be buried haphazardly, anywhere, on a clifftop overlooking the Channel which he had failed so dismally to guard. Another story is that the body was carried northwards to Waltham Abbey, Harold's own foundation, and buried there.

But, as with so many elements in the enigma of Hastings, nothing is sure.

Epilogue

The story is told. England had been won by the invader after a day of frightful slaughter and mayhem, and as we leave William drinking his champagne, with Heaven knows what thoughts coursing through his exhausted mind, the new England which his victory created was about to be born. But that is a fresh story altogether.

The overwhelming fact about William's conquest is that out of the plotting and machinations (including a welter of events of which there is now no trace or hint), the savageries, and a single battle on the sloping meadow of Senlac, there emerged a kingdom which was to grow in strength and influence for 900 years; until, that is, its Empire crumbled and it found itself searching for a new role to play. William was, in truth, the father of a country which until the mid-1970s was the biggest single influence in the making of the world of today. And there were plain signs as the twentieth century rolled on that the wheel of history was about to complete a full circle since 1066 – that the descendants of the Anglo-Normans, still free from any intervening military invasion, were going back across the Channel, perhaps to lead the Europe from which William and his knights hailed to the first real unity it had ever seen.

I am acutely aware that not all who read this present work will accept its recital of the prelude to the Conquest or endorse many of the deductions made therein. This is not surprising considering that more arguments and quarrels about what really happened have persisted throughout centuries of increasing confusion, exaggeration and stubborn conceits, than about any other episode in the history of man. There are two chief reasons for the continuing excitement. They are, first, the magnitude of the effects of the Conquest and, second, the scope for theorizing and imagining permitted by the absence of so much important evidence, and the contradiction and haziness enveloping that which is known.

However, the dominating personality of the chief protagonist, William of Normandy, shines clearly and unequivocally through the haze. To a far lesser degree, so does something of the character of the man he defeated, although any student of the fateful clash between the two men cannot help but yearn for even a few more scraps of information about him. The third figure, Edward the Confessor, is well documented, but he remains elusive and mysterious simply because he was obviously that kind of man.

Fortunately, actual pictures of these three characters in our story have survived to show clearly what they looked like physically. This valuable evidence is to be found in coins struck while they were alive. These tokens are surprisingly consistent considering that the art of coin making was still primitive and also that those struck for the two English kings were produced in various parts of the country by men who had mostly to work without ever seeing their subjects. The coins of William all reflect a man with a hard, cruel mouth, and somewhat saturnine – what we should expect.

Those of Harold, on the other hand, depict a man of bright, blithe and alert mien, with no sign of fat or of loose muscles at the age of 44 when he became king. Volatile – that is the word which crosses the mind as one looks closely at these likenesses of Harold; one or two moneyers have caught what might very well have been the authentic personality by perching the crown on Harold's head lightly and jauntily. The number of his coins is necessarily sparse because he reigned for less than 11 months and was so perpetually on the move meeting one challenge after another that moneyer or artist could not have had many opportunities to do his work. Incidentally, the coins of Harold (certainly all those in the splendid Hunterian and Coats Collection at the University of Glasgow) show a face fringed with a trimmed beard. This is superficially not a world-shaking fact, but it has a deeper significance than would appear because it contradicts the Bayeux Tapestry and provides modest additional ammunition for those who do not accept the Tapestry as a form of holy testament. A further point is that the Tapestry also depicts William as clean shaven, whereas all his coins show him bearded.

The third royal figure, Edward the Confessor, is also shown bearded in all the coins struck during his reign of 24 years between

1042 and 1066, and this squares with the likenesses of him in the Tapestry. Here again the moneyers are unanimous; they show him as a slight scholarly figure and they keep up faithfully with his ageing. He is boylike, almost, in 1042 and wispily elderly in the coins struck during the final years of his reign.

One of the most recent of his coins to be unearthed was a silver penny picked up by Geoffrey Lythe while he was clearing stones with a bowser on a short stretch of Roman road in Catterton Road, Tadcaster, nine miles south of York, on 20 September 1969. The excavating was being done, under the inspection of historians, for the laying of pipes to carry natural gas inland from the floor of the North Sea. Many enthusiasts hoped the coin had been dropped by one of Harold's Housecarls during the phenomenal ride north to confront Harald Hardrada and Tostig, especially since Harold and his men must have used this particular stretch of Roman road. Alas, the odds are heavily against this being so, for the coin had been struck by a local moneyer, Angrim of York, and Harold's men were riding from the south and would scarcely have been carrying northern coins. But the enthusiasts do not give up readily. They say that the silver penny might just as easily have fallen from the purse or pocket of a Housecarl who had fought at the Battle of Stamford Bridge and was riding back south to fight at Senlac. Whatever its origin, the penny was declared treasure trove and an inquest was arranged by Tadcaster County Police. The verdict was that it belonged to the Earl of Halifax, on whose land it had been found. Lord Halifax generously gave it back to its finder, Mr Lythe, who then equally generously handed it over to the Yorkshire Museum in York. He was paid a bounty of £6 for it.

As for the Battle of Hastings itself, so little is known about it that one marvels at the plenitude and persuasiveness of the accounts which have been produced about it, one after the other, since the Middle Ages. They vary remarkably in detail, scope and style according to the imagination and selectivity of the writers, but they do conform broadly to a kind of approved version of the battle which has been built up. This should by no means be taken to prove that the accepted version is the correct one. On the contrary, it is almost certain that this version strays quite a long way from the truth. It is founded upon one contemporary account by the biassed and often demonstrably unreliable Norman scribe, William of Poitiers, the pictures in the Tapestry and a few later versions written within approximately 100 years of the event and themselves based, but with elaborations and distortions, upon William of Poitiers. Consequently, the more enthusiastically a modern writer goes into detail about the battle the more likely he is to be wrong, like a lost traveller seeking to find his destination on the basis of not one but several sets of faulty directions.

I do not for a moment pretend that the account given in this work avoids all such errors and pitfalls. But it might be closer to the mark of accuracy because it has been severely restricted to describing those episodes which almost certainly did happen or may be considered as highly probable in view of indications in the prime sources, from observation of the terrain, and the existence of such landmarks as Telham Hill, the London–Hastings road and Battle Abbey. For example, the incident so clearly shown in the Tapestry of Duke William raising his visor to dispel the alarming rumour that he had been killed can hardly be dismissed as having been totally imagined by the creators of the Tapestry. I believe this interlude happened precisely as depicted. As noted in our narrative, the death of a commander in battle was usually a decisive disaster for his side and the alert and practical William would act promptly and effectively to show that this had not happened. Again, the fact that a hillock is still discernible in just the spot where one would expect to find it offers some confirmation of the chastening incident in which bolting English levies were annihilated after breaking out from Harold's shield-wall. Further, the spot where Harold raised his standards and fought and was killed is identified almost to a pinpoint by the situation of the High Altar of Battle Abbey, built by William's order to commemorate his victory, and this item of identification helps enormously in tracing the rest of the English line on Senlac ridge.

It is a pity indeed that so much evidence which must have existed after the battle has been destroyed or is lost deeply beneath the accumulation of centuries of urbanizing development. Little more than 100 yards from the spot where Harold fell stands today a social hall (dedicated to the memory of young local Englishmen who died in two world wars in the twentieth century) in which Sussex youth may be seen dancing away their Saturday nights. The modern version of the track along which Duke William and his men marched to battle in 1066 is lined today with terraces of Victorian and later villas. The community of Battle has spread all

over the site of one end of the English line and Harold's immediate
left rear. But the battlefield itself remains more or less unchanged,
offering an exciting view to the imaginative visitor. Parts of Senlac
meadow are still being farmed, and cattle graze on the lower slopes
below the battlefront where all the slaughter was done.

Offsetting the vagueness and incompleteness of our knowledge
of the battle is the fact of its singularly decisive consequences. It
yielded the whole of England to William – an undoubted surprise
to him as a realist who had expected a far different and more
difficult turn of events after the victory. No conqueror before him
had ever gained England at one stroke. Belgae, Romans, Vikings
and all the others had had to fight one hard battle after another to
annex chunks of territory as they advanced, and the resources of
most of them had been exhausted long before they had penetrated
from one shore to another. There is no doubt that the wary William
had expected a similarly tough ordeal after Senlac. Instead of
marching boldly upon London as soon as he had rested and
regrouped his force after the battle, he turned eastwards along
the coast to capture Dover, which fell to him without a fight even
though it was a manned citadel, and even then he did not strike
directly into London, the kingdom's heart. He ventured slowly
north-east from Dover in the direction of the capital, plundering and
destroying as he went, and eventually halted at Southwark on
the south bank of the Thames. Then he turned west. He evidently
concluded that London was too tough a nut to crack with his
depleted strength and accordingly resolved to isolate it until it fell
to him of its own volition. He marched south-west as far as Winchester, now the second city of England, and again he received
surrender without a fight. Even the cautious William must have
reached the conclusion by this time that his victory at Senlac had
been total. He now turned north and eventually reached the
Thames at Wallingford, 40 miles upstream from London, and was
given conclusive evidence that there was in fact to be no massed
resistance to him. Stigand, the Archbishop of Canterbury, met him
at Wallingford and offered him submission, and Stigand was
quickly followed by the rest of the formerly powerful figures in the
kingdom. William did not have to draw the sword again to complete
his formal conquest; his troubles with insurrectionists and guerillas
were to come later, to plague him for the rest of his life. He was
crowned King of England in Westminster Abbey on Christmas Day,

just a year after Edward the Confessor had died and Harold had been crowned in the same edifice, and only three months after he had landed at Pevensey.

Two principal reasons accounted for this remarkable triumph. One was that England at that time was not a unified kingdom under a truly national ruler; it was not even as closely knit as it had been under Edward the Confessor and certainly not as unified as under Alfred the Great, a century and a half earlier. The other reason was that the House of Godwin perished utterly on the field at Senlac, and nobody was left who was either willing or able to take the place of Harold and his brothers in resisting William. The only possible surviving challengers were the brothers Edwin and Morcar, and they had lately been given such a thrashing by Harald Hardrada in the north that whatever spunk they might have had (and their records both before and after the Conquest indicated that they were not over-endowed with either courage or determination) had been dissipated. After a weak flicker of energy when they talked about setting up the juvenile Edgar Atheling as a royal rival to William but did nothing concrete towards accomplishing this, they weakly joined everybody else in accepting William. The final capitulation came at Berkhamsted. Thereafter, Edwin and Morcar never figured again in national affairs. They were treated with contempt by William until they died in separate obscurities.

One final thought. All of us who are interested in building up a substantial and accurate story of the avalanche of events immediately before the Conquest can feel only frustration at the one-sidedness and dubiousness of written and pictorial evidence from the Norwegian and Norman sides and the deviousness and scantness of detail which detracts from what is available from the English side. This is compounded by the truly astonishing lack of tangible mementoes of William's invasion, Harold's reaction to it and their climatic meeting at Senlac. Even the Bayeux Tapestry, finest relic of all, is not complete. An unknown length of it, at the end, is missing. It concludes in frayed remnants after a panel picturing the flight of defeated English survivors of Senlac towards the Andredsweald. Nobody knows how much more of the story has been lost to neglect and the ravages of the elements during nine centuries, and it would be of vast help to inquirers if by some miracle even some fragments of the lost embroidery were found again. Probably more exciting and revealing would be the discovery of a picture, drawing, object or manuscript – even a sentence or two of contemporary or near-contemporary writing – to illuminate the English side of the story of Senlac.

Does any such evidence still exist today? If so, will it ever be located? One can only hope. It is not really such a slender hope. After all, one of the finest examples of the work of Saxon gold-smiths and metal workers – Alfred's Jewel – was not found until about 800 years after it had been created. It was unearthed by chance in a field behind the rectory at North Newton, Somerset, in 1693. It had lain underneath a house which was being demolished at that time on the lands of Sir Thomas Wrothe, Lord of the Manor. Its name and authenticity come from a Saxon inscription in Roman lettering – *Alfred Mec Heht Gewyrcan* (Alfred had me made) – fortified by some typically Saxon fine gold filigree. The Jewel, which now lies in permanent sanctuary within the Ashmolean Museum in Oxford, is only two and a half inches long. Who can say that, somewhere, does not lie some equally small and en-lightening relic of William's invasion and the Enigma of Hastings?

Appendix A

Professor de Bouard reported (in a personal account to the author) that Mathilda's tomb, in the choir of the private chapel of the *Abbaye aux Dames*, was damaged during the French Revolution. It was restored in 1819 and while the rehabilitation was being accomplished, an inventory of the dried bones of the queen was made by Dr Dominel, a surgeon attached to the Hospital of Caen. The bones were laid out in a small lead coffin which was then placed inside a stone sarcophagus. Two of four vellum copies of Dr Dominel's report and an account of the re-internment were put into bottles, one of which was laid inside the lead coffin and the other inside the sarcophagus.

In 1960 the tomb was reopened by a joint decision of the Mayor of Caen, the regional Keeper of Buildings in France and the Chief Architect of Historical Documents. Professor de Bouard was in attendance as Regional Director of Historic Antiquities in charge of the administration of archeological excavations. 'The monument put up in 1819 was very ugly and detracted from the Roman choir of the Chapel, and this was why the tomb was reopened in 1960,' he said. 'The decision was to remove it and to put into the tiling of the floor the tombstone which marked the first resting-place of Queen Mathilda constructed in 1083 and bearing a very nice inscription.'

The sarcophagus and inner lead coffin were duly found under the monument. When Professor de Bouard opened the coffin he found the remains of Mathilda just as they had been described by Dr Dominel in 1819. 'An anthropological examination of these remains was made,' said the Professor. 'It shows that Mathilda was a really tiny person, 1.46 metres tall, and thin.'

The remains were thoroughly dehydrated and rendered into a condition of preservation. Then they were placed in an urn of rustless steel filled with a gas conducive to permanent preservation. They now rest in the new tomb.

One interesting sidelight to the history of the queen's remains is that the two vellum copies of Dr Dominel's report which were sealed in bottles and laid inside the sarcophagus and lead coffin in 1819 were found in 1960 to have disintegrated. The bottles contained nothing but a liquid resembling dirty water. An examination made at the bacteriological laboratory of the University of Caen disclosed that the liquid was the product of microbe activity, which had caused the total dissolution of the vellum. Luckily, one other of the four copies made of the Dominel report survived in the archives of the Department of Calvados.

Appendix B

It is an interesting exercise to cause one's mind to flit back over some nine centuries and picture just a few prosaic, practical examples of how men's minds and lives were cramped by ignorance. People knew nothing, comparatively, about the universe around them so that a comet streaking across the sky or an eclipse bringing unnatural darkness baffled them; and because nature and the elements seemed mostly to be working so cruelly against them such happenings were automatically adjudged to be portents of coming disaster or punishment. The chronicles of Anglo-Saxon England abound in examples of this kind of fearful interpretation of phenomena which later generations have come not only to understand but to be able to forecast to within minute fractions of a second. They knew little about the symptoms, treatment and cure of disease and a disablement such as blindness or defective eyesight, fits, or even an infection, had to be borne as an inevitable and irremediable affliction. A catastrophe such as a stroke or the onset of a devouring disease could neither be identified nor cured and was accepted as a portent of certain and usually speedy death. Bubonic and smallpox diseases were frequent scourges. One, perhaps two, people in a settlement in England or northern Europe would be found to have been stricken. Men had found to their cost that such diseases spread quickly and horribly. So the first detected victims were exiled outside the stockade of the settlement, among the strips or furlongs ('furrow longs' as the Anglo-Saxons called the rectangles of cultivated lands divided by lines of earth and stones). The sufferers were fed from a distance. Occasionally one person would eventually recover and a miracle would be proclaimed but mostly the afflicted ones died because nobody knew how to tend them; and often the isolation would have been made too late. An epidemic would develop, more and more people would die, and the chroniclers would record the doleful news : 'Such a malady fell upon men that very nearly every other person was in the sorriest plight and down with fever; it was so malignant that many died from the disease.'

Mortality rates were so high that modern calculators believe that in an average village or settlement on both sides of the English Channel during the eleventh century it would take about two years to add one person to the local population. This is not surprising since a natural disaster such as flood, drought, fire or a destructive tempest would claim many victims and one such catastrophe usually meant hunger and famine for months among the survivors; two successive catastrophes often meant the complete destruction of a settlement. Men were so powerless against the excesses of nature, having pitifully few of the defences which the spread of knowledge and technical inventiveness later enabled them to use, that it is not surprising there should have been such an abundance of strange superstitions and unreasoning fears. Even privileged and superior secular leaders like Anselm, Cuthbert of Lindisfarne, and the Venerable Bede were beset and hobbled by many of the widespread mental and psychological infirmities and handicaps of their times, and their deeds and writings are all the more to be marvelled at on that account.

Woman as a whole had a harder and more humdrum life than their men. Apart from the high born and the more high-spirited women, who were often treated with unusual respect and enjoyed some authority, they were more the chattels than the partners of their menfolk. A woman's role was principally to serve man as he demanded and within certain strict limitations to be used as he pleased. But there *were* limits. A sexual assault upon a resisting woman, or rape, brought a penalty of immediate castration of the offender in Anglo-Saxon England.

Scholars who have examined surviving poems and ballads of the era in England, Normandy and Scandinavia have found them to be notably prim and mostly devoted to masculine military prowess, although some do reflect warmth of feeling between men and women. They often express the yearnings of women for comradeship and they dwell upon woman's sadness at the long and frequent absence of a warrior husband. This early poetry rarely goes into details of sexual love, but some evidence has been found of the existence of a lusty bawdiness which might be regarded as the forerunner of the kind of thing so much enjoyed by the later Elizabethans. Thus, in his biography of Edward the Confessor published in 1970, Professor Barlow includes two eleventh-century riddles in which *double entendre* is used adroitly, amusingly and obscenely. One riddle asks for the identity of an object described as follows :

I am the world's wonder, for I make women happy.
I am well set up, stand in a bed,
Have a roughish root. Rarely (though it happens)
A churl's daughter more daring than the rest
– and lovelier – lays hold of me,
Rushes my red top, wrenches at my head,
And lays me in the larder. She learns soon enough,
The curly-headed creature who clamps me so,
Of my meeting with her : moist is her eye !

The answer, unexpectedly, is – an onion.

Appendix C

William of Poitiers states that William was delayed a month while awaiting a favourable southerly wind at the Dives estuary. While this chronicler is suspect on many points there seems no reason to question this particular statement, especially as it is inferentially confirmed by entries in the Anglo-Saxon Chronicle and elsewhere which indicate that William intended to invade much earlier than he did.

It is generally believed that William eventually sailed for Pevensey from St Valery on the night of 27 September after recovering from the disaster of the storm which fell upon him soon after he had left the Dives. Now, an entry in the *Carmen de Hastingae Proelis* written in 1067 (very soon indeed after the event) and attributed to the highly respected authority of Guy, Archbishop of Amiens, states that William waited again for a favourable wind a period of 'three times five days' (*ter quinque dies*) after putting into St Valery for refuge after the storm. Adding these 15 days to the month spent by William at the Dives estuary we get a period of approximately 45 days between his first departure from Normandy and his landfall at Pevensey. We should probably add something like a week to this period for extra delay caused by the storm and time used by William to dispose of his dead, repair smashed boats and for his troops to regain their equilibrium and their spirit. We thereby reach the date of about 6 August as the moment of William's first readiness.

The matter is engagingly discussed by Professor Douglas in his *William the Conqueror* (Eyre and Spottiswoode, 1964].

Bibliography

The Bayeux Tapestry is, of course, the prime source of information about the Norman invasion of England and the battle which followed. Many reproductions are available. Two which proved invaluable in the writing of this book were:

1 *The Bayeux Tapestry* (Phaidon, 1965), which contains some magnificent reproductions in colour of Tapestry panels and also a series of essays by experts about the Tapestry's production, history and meaning.

2 Eric Maclagen, *The Bayeux Tapestry* (Penguin, rev. ed. 1953), which is less ambitious in scope but contains much shrewdly-reasoned information about the Tapestry.

One other source of a different kind is outstanding. It is Douglas, David C., and Greenway, George W., *English Historical Documents* (Eyre and Spottiswoode, 1968). It is a costly book but worth every penny paid for it. Herein are to be found not only ample passages of all the relevant chronicles, but also letters, writs and other basic documents throwing light upon the history of England between 1042 and 1189.

Other valuable works consulted include:

Anglo-Saxon Chronicle, The, trans. G. N. Garmonsway (Dent, 1960).

Amiens, Guy of, *Carmen de Hastingensi Proelio,* in F. Michel, *Chroniques Anglo-Normandes,* vol. III (Rouen, E. Frere, 1836–40).

Bede, the Venerable, *Ecclesiastical History of England,* trans. Dr J. A. Giles (Henry J. Bohn, London, 1849).

Clare, Osbert of, *The Letters of Osbert of Clare,* ed. E. W. Williamson (Oxford, 1929).

Durham, Simeon of, *Opera Omnia,* ed. T. Arnold (Rolls Series, 1882–5).

Eadmer, *Vita Anselmi,* trans. and ed. R. W. Southern (Nelson, 1962).

Huntingdon, Henry of, *Historia Anglorum*, ed. T. Arnold (Rolls Series, 1879).

Malmesbury, William of, *A History of the Kings of England*, trans. Rev. John Sharpe (Longman, Hunt, Rees, Orme and Brown, London, 1815).

——, ——, *Vita Wulfstani*, ed. R. R. Darlington (Royal Historical Society, Camden, 1928).

Orkeyingers Saga, trans. Alexander Burt Taylor (Oliver and Boyd, 1938).

Poitiers, William of, 'The Deeds of William, Duke of the Normans and King of the English', in *English Historical Documents* (see above).

Snorri, Sturlasen, *Heimskringla*, trans. Samuel Laing (Norrena Society, 1906).

Vitalis, Ordericus, *Ecclesiastical History*, 4 vols., trans. T. Forester (Bohn's Antiquarian Library, London, 1853–6).

Worcester, Florence of, *Chronicon ex Chronicis*, trans. J. Stevenson (*Church Historians of England*, Vol. II, London, 1853).

General

Baker, Timothy, *The Normans* (Macmillan, New York, 1966).

Barclay, C. N., *Battle 1066* (Dent, 1966).

Barlow, Frank, *Edward the Confessor* (Eyre and Spottiswoode, 1970).

Blair, Peter Hunter, *An Introduction to Anglo-Saxon England* (Cambridge, 1962).

Bloch, Marc, *Feudal Society*, vol. I, trans. L. A. Manyon (Routledge and Kegan Paul, 1971).

Bouard, Michel de, *Guillaume le Conquerant* (Paris, 1958).

Brooks, F. W., *The Battle of Stamford Bridge* (East Yorkshire Local History Society, 1956).

Butler, Denis, *1066 – The Story of a Year* (G. P. Putnam's Sons, New York, 1966).

Codrington, Thomas, *Roman Roads in Britain* (Sheldon Press, 1928).

Douglas, David C., *William the Conqueror* (Eyre and Spottiswoode, 1964).

Freeman, E. A., *The History of the Norman Conquest of England*, 5 vols and Index vol. (Oxford, 1870–1879).

Fuller, J. F. C., *Julius Caesar – Man, Soldier and Tyrant* (Eyre and Spottiswoode, 1965).

Gloag, John, *2,000 Years of England* (Cassell, 1952).

Grierson, Philip, *A Visit by Earl Harold to Flanders in 1056* (English Historical Review, 1936).

Jane, L. C., *Asser's Life of King Alfred* (Cooper Square Publisher, New York, 1966).

Jerrold, Douglas, *Introduction to the History of England* (Collins, 1949).

Johnson, Paul, *The Offshore Islanders: England's People from Roman Occupation to the Present* (Weidenfeld and Nicolson 1972).

Kelly, Amy, *Eleanor of Aquitaine* (Vintage Books, New York, 1950).

Lamb, H. H., *The Changing Climate* (Methuen, 1972).

Lemmon, C. H., *The Field of Hastings* (Budd and Gillatt, 2nd ed. 1960).

Linklater, Eric, *The Conquest of England* (Doubleday, New York, 1966).

Maitland, F. W., *Domesday Book and Beyond* (Collins, 1961).

Milton, John, *History of England* (Printed for James Allestry at the Rose and Crown, St Paul's Churchyard, 1670).

Muntz, Hope, *The Golden Warrior* (Scribner's, New York, 1951).

Oman, Charles, *A History of the Art of War in the Middle Ages*, vol. I (Burt and Franklin, New York, 1924).

Palmer, V. E., and M. L., *A History of Earls Barton* (Steeple Press, 1970).

Plummer, Charles, *Life and Times of Alfred* (Haskell House, New York, 1970).

Quennell, Marjorie and C. H. B., *Everyday Life in Roman and Anglo-Saxon Times* (Batsford, 1959).

Stenton, F. M., *Anglo-Saxon England* (Oxford, 1943).

Trevelyan, G. M., *English Social History* (Longmans Green, 1945).

Vine, Francis, T., *Caesar in Kent* (Turnbull and Spears, 1886).

Williamson, J. A., *The English Channel* (Collins, 1959).

Index

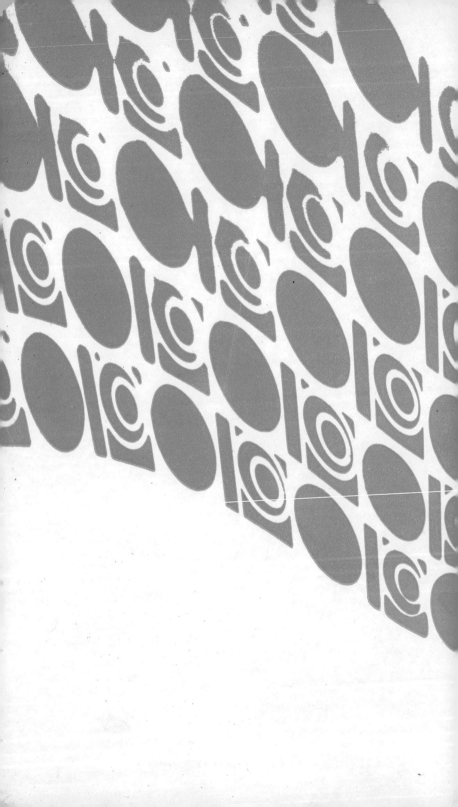